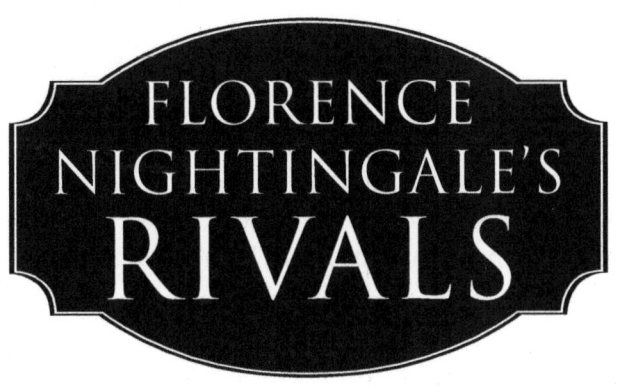

For my granddaughter Evie, who always makes me smile and has granted me the gift of never being able to say no.

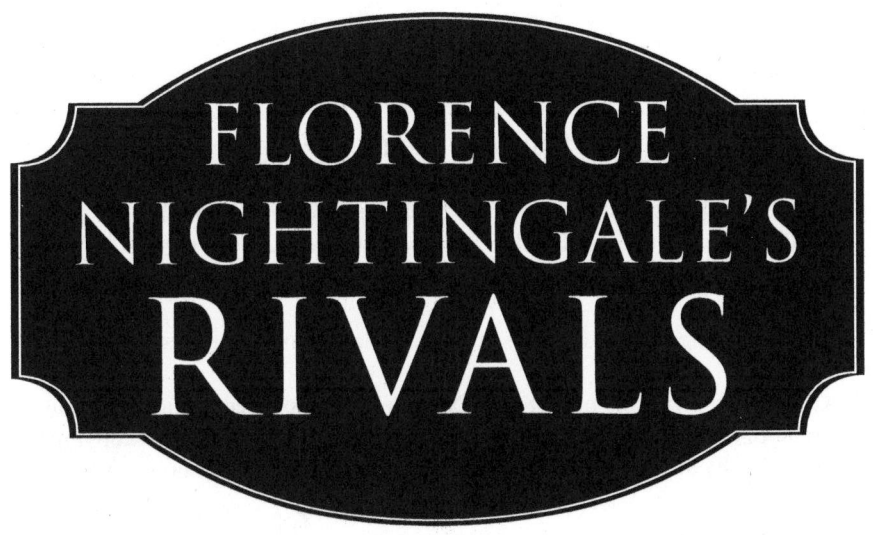

# FLORENCE NIGHTINGALE'S RIVALS

## NURSING THROUGH THE CRIMEA

## LOUISE WYATT

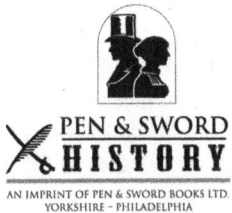

PEN & SWORD **HISTORY**

AN IMPRINT OF PEN & SWORD BOOKS LTD.
YORKSHIRE - PHILADELPHIA

First published in Great Britain in 2024 by
**PEN AND SWORD HISTORY**
An imprint of
Pen & Sword Books Ltd
Yorkshire – Philadelphia

Copyright © Louise Wyatt, 2024

ISBN 978 1 39900 665 1

The right of Louise Wyatt to be identified as Author of this work has been asserted by her in accordance with the Copyright, Designs and Patents Act 1988.

A CIP catalogue record for this book is available from the British Library.

All rights reserved. No part of this book may be reproduced or transmitted in any form or by any means, electronic or mechanical including photocopying, recording or by any information storage and retrieval system, without permission from the Publisher in writing.

Typeset in Times New Roman 12/16 by
SJmagic DESIGN SERVICES, India.
Printed and bound in the UK by CPI Group (UK) Ltd.

Pen & Sword Books Limited incorporates the imprints of Atlas, Archaeology, Aviation, Discovery, Family History, Fiction, History, Maritime, Military, Military Classics, Politics, Select, Transport, True Crime, Air World, Frontline Publishing, Leo Cooper, Remember When, Seaforth Publishing, The Praetorian Press, Wharncliffe Local History, Wharncliffe Transport, Wharncliffe True Crime and White Owl.

*For a complete list of Pen & Sword titles please contact*
**PEN & SWORD BOOKS LIMITED**
George House, Units 12 & 13, Beevor Street, Off Pontefract Road,
Barnsley, South Yorkshire, S71 1HN, England
E-mail: enquiries@pen-and-sword.co.uk
Website: www.pen-and-sword.co.uk

or

PEN AND SWORD BOOKS
1950 Lawrence Rd, Havertown, PA 19083, USA
E-mail: uspen-and-sword@casematepublishers.com
Website: www.penandswordbooks.com

# Contents

Acknowledgements ................................................................. vi

Introduction ......................................................................... vii

Chapter 1    Nursing from Antiquity to Victorian England ............. 1

Chapter 2    Crimean Call to Nursing Arms ................................ 26

Chapter 3    Sister Mary Francis Bridgeman:
             short biography to 1854 ............................................ 53

Chapter 4    Betsy Cadwaladyr: short biography to 1854 ............. 58

Chapter 5    Florence Nightingale: short biography to 1854 ........ 64

Chapter 6    Relationships in the Crimea .................................... 79

Chapter 7    Going Home ....................................................... 128

Appendix 1   Adapted from Maslow's Heirarchy of Needs ......... 142

Appendix 2   Scutari & Koulali Hospitals January 1855 ............. 143

Notes ................................................................................. 144

Bibliography ....................................................................... 158

Index .................................................................................. 175

# Acknowledgements

WITH MANY THANKS to Bet Melville, fluent speaker/reader/writer of the Welsh language, who translated many bits of historical information, allowing me to add much context to the story of Betsy Cadwaladyr. Also, to William Powell, for the help with everything to do with maths, graphs and statistics.

# Introduction

*FLORENCE NIGHTINGALE'S RIVALS: Nursing Through the Crimea* was born from researching my previous *History of Nursing* book, where I came across some interesting personality dynamics during the Crimean War (1854 – 1856) between two very strong characters in the form of Betsy Cadwaladyr and Mother Mary Francis Bridgeman, the Mother Superior of the nursing Irish Sisters of Mercy. There were too many stories to be told then but finally, this book formed to tell the stories of these two nurses who served in the Crimean War.

These two women jumped out at me but are not well known to the general public or the history of the Crimea. I discuss them alongside Florence Nightingale to show the comparison of their work and how, by the end of the war, they had both earned respect from Nightingale; although best friends they could never be. It is worth noting that for this book, I take the Crimean War from March 1854, when Britain and France joined the war that had erupted between Russia and Turkey in October 1853.

With regard to nursing, the Crimean War is synonymous with the name and person of Florence Nightingale, who was contracted by the government in October 1854 to lead a small group of female nurses to assist the medical men in caring for the wounded and diseased soldiers in what was turning out to be an unmitigated disaster. However, things went a lot deeper than that; my research highlighted many deep-rooted biases, mainly religion, ethnicity and social class. Whilst many of these belief systems are anathema to us today, they are what Victorian Britain lived, breathed and functioned on.

Logistically, any form of army medical/nursing care and medical supplies in 1854 was a ridiculous mish-mash of outdated knowledge, bad planning and a tragic misunderstanding of the needs of the military. In February 1854 the Director General of the Army Medical Department was Dr Andrew Smith, who was tasked with supplying and preparing the army with medical stores and personnel. After forty years of peace and with his meagre staff of two medical officers, four clerks and no one with experience of what was needed to supply adequate medical staff and stores, Smith found no official documents or guidance to help him build upon, but he still submitted what was required purely from his own judgement. He organised a reconnaissance to assess the situation with a surgical contact in Constantinople, which received no support from the military. He told the War Office in April 1854 that a hospital corps of 800 men were needed to become ambulance drivers, stretcher-bearers and orderlies, but those the War Office finally bothered sending out in July 1854 were too elderly or drunk, as we see in Nightingale's and Betsy's description of these men later in the book.

It is not a surprise that Dr Smith was made – rather unfairly – one of the scapegoats by the government and by Florence Nightingale at the end of the war, of all that had gone wrong. Coincidentally, he also came from a working-class background and had worked hard to get to where he was. Even the initial nursing arrangements did not go to plan. Sidney Herbert, Secretary at War, allegedly acting on a supposed letter from Nightingale's guardian Sir Charles Bracebridge explaining that Nightingale would not be averse to more nurses, arranged for another party of volunteer nurses to go out to the Crimea.

It was with this second group that Betsy Cadwaladyr and Mother Bridgeman went out in December 1854. When they arrived, Nightingale lost her temper – especially with her friend Sidney Herbert – as this had not been planned or discussed; she had no room

## Introduction

for them and as she did not know what to do with them, she sent them to stay at the British Ambassador's residence. Betsy disliked Nightingale before she had even met her and Mother Bridgeman demanded her nuns had their own religious space or they would leave.

The distaste at not having any work, let alone no nursing duties, allocated to them began to breed discontent and not just amongst the women this book is focusing on, but from the Lady Nurses, too; the wealthy ladies of society that, although considered management material, could not be paid as only the working classes received a salary. What must be remembered, though, is that Florence Nightingale herself was under immense pressure from authorities such as the government and the medical men and had constraints she had to stay within, especially regarding numbers of nursing personnel. And Nightingale was determined to live by the rules, something Besty did not always believe in, while the only rules Mother Bridgeman agreed to were those of her religious order.

The Irish Sisters of Mercy were perhaps, at the beginning anyway, the ones with the longest history and experience of hands-on nursing and administration of actual clinical care. They had experience with nursing cholera amongst their local communities, which was endemic at the beginning of the Crimean War, with Mother Bridgeman bringing her skill with a cramp-relieving poultice to the soldiers. They also bought with them their Careful Nursing philosophy, which had been a founding charter of the Sisters of Mercy's founder, Catherine McAuley. Today's nurses will recognise it as holistic care and find it in the hospice movement's Total Pain model. Florence Nightingale has been known to mention Careful Nursing in her *Notes on Nursing* and *Notes on Hospitals* books, with no acknowledgement to the Sisters of Mercy, although there are studies exerting the fact that Careful Nursing itself is a skill across the board and innate to nursing, not just exclusive to the Sisters of Mercy. The nuns also had to contend with the politics of the Irish 'problem'. This is examined in more detail later in the book, but the Irish Famine, the general mistrust of the Irish people and the unwanted resurgence of high-ranking positions in the Catholic church in the mid-nineteenth century have led to the work of the Sisters of Mercy being unknown, overlooked and largely ignored in their nursing efforts of the Crimean War.

Careful Nursing evolved from these early Irish nurses, with McAuley reiterating the importance of easing distress and comfort of the patient.[1] This was not a new thing *per se*; Hippocrates recognised the importance of holistic care in the fifth century and understood the need to care for the well-being and inner peace of the mind and body as well as the physical.[2] One of the 1948 founding constitutions of the World Health Organisation states 'Health is a state of complete physical, mental and social well-being and not merely the absence of disease or infirmity'. In nursing today, spiritual care without the religious connotations (McAuley first practised this form of nursing as a secular activity) is recognised as an integral part of delivering holistic nursing care, whether you are a newly qualified or advanced nurse. It is about responding to the emotional, spiritual needs of a patient when facing illness, trauma or mental health problems and the need for sensitive listening; the whole was bought together in 1964 by Dame Cicely Saunders, the founder of the hospice movement we know today as Total Pain, incorporating physical symptoms, mental distress, social problems and emotional difficulties.[3] Therefore, although the need to comfort has been felt and explained in various ways over millennia, McAuley bought it back from the darkness left by the Reformation 300 years earlier, with the Visitation of the Sick Rule No.8 stating 'Great tenderness must be employed … to relieve distress first … to promote the cleanliness, ease and comfort of the Patient'.[4]

Not only did this careful nursing philosophy spread to other continents with the foundations of new Sisters of Mercy convents, it was also taken to the Crimea by Mother Bridgeman. It appears to have been successful; just before Mother Bridgeman departed for home from the Crimea with her Sisters, Nightingale 'took notes of our manner of nursing which Rev Mother [Bridgeman] explained to her as she hoped someone might profit of it.'[5] Although, personality-wise,

*Introduction*

Bridgeman and Nightingale did not get on particularly well, Nightingale was impressed with the Sisters' careful nursing system, even incorporating it into her *Notes on Nursing* published in 1859: '… the exact value of particular remedies and modes of treatment is by no means ascertained, while there is universal experience as to the extreme importance of careful nursing in determining the issue of disease.'[6] Also in her *Notes on Hospitals* in 1863, when making recommendations to the government: 'And as everybody knows, a patient may often be saved by careful nursing when everything else will fail.'[7]

Interestingly, there is no acknowledgement to the Sisters of Mercy around these statements. In more recent times, Professor Lynn McDonald has questioned the plaudits of the careful nursing system used in the Crimea and its relevance to the Sisters of Mercy. In her 2014 paper 'Florence Nightingale and Irish Nursing', McDonald criticises Dr Meehan's assertion that the Irish Sisters were '… recognised as skilled nurses and had attained brilliant prestige in nursing', with Dr Meehan herself quoting from Volume III of one of the most respected history of nursing's four-volume reference work by Nutting & Dock, published in 1907 (vols I and II) and Dock in 1912 (vols III and IV). McDonald ascertains that this was a brief reference to McAuley alone, but in Dock's original reference it actually reads: 'The order of the Sisters of Mercy, founded in Dublin, in 1831, early attained brilliant prestige in nursing.'[8] McDonald compares this brief reference in Volume III to the whole of Volume II being dedicated to Florence Nightingale's nursing, as well as other religious nursing[9].

Thirteen years later however, Dock – in her book *A Short History of Nursing* – does give more thought to Irish nursing, going back as far as the seventh century and how the Irish nuns had an ancient but progressive tradition of passing on their nursing skills down through monasteries over time.[10] However, Nightingale was much better known in the British public eye in 1907 (and still alive!) whereas the Sisters of Mercy were not and their achievements, as well as their nursing stories of the Crimea, were not known until later years. This was partly political and partly the wishes of the Sisters themselves; they did not want the glory or admiration, just the chance to go back to their work. The three Sisters of Mercy's extant diaries of Bridgeman, Croke and Doyle were not published until after their deaths; this will be discussed later in the book.

McDonald quite rightly states that the careful nursing system in the Crimea did not directly influence Nightingale's work post-war;[11] she must have considered it when writing her *Notes* books mentioned earlier, but Nightingale was more concerned with the theory and statistics of what she had witnessed and putting them into sanitary reforms.

This book therefore aims to look at the work of these two women in addition to Nightingale. Thanks to Nightingale's social position and her contacts in government, this is who and what is generally known about nursing in the Crimea. Nightingale most definitely had a very difficult job and a rather difficult position in getting things right when out in the Crimea, but looking a bit further from this shows us some other interesting stories and events.

Betsy, although one of the working-class/hospital nurses, had a strong faith and did not drink, unlike Charles Dickens' Sarah Gamp characters of her fellow travellers to the Crimea. She got very defensive when classed as one of them, but what cannot be denied is how hardworking she was. Her autobiography – albeit occasionally questioned for its complete accuracy – is the only record of a working-class woman in the Crimean War. It is used largely here to form the chapter of Betsy, along with the diaries still extant to us today of the three Sisters of Mercy (Bridgeman, Doyle and Croker), as well as the many letters of Nightingale.

Interestingly, there are many written accounts of statistics, experiences and recommendations by the surgeons and doctors on the battlefield too, many of which have thankfully been put on the www.archive.org website and make for interesting reading. I have also utilised the literary account of Fanny Taylor, one of the Lady Nurses who also wrote about her experiences and gave some interesting

## Introduction

insights to events; one can almost feel her frustration at not having work to do when she also arrived with the second party of nurses.

A myriad of articles, studies and biographies of Florence Nightingale exist and after much reviewing, I decided to stick with Sir Edward Cook's 1913 original biography, commissioned by Nightingale's family after she had passed away and still considered to be the best. I dabbled with Ida O'Malley's 1931 account up until Nightingale left the Crimea, as she had access to some family papers that Cook did not, and finally, a scrupulously researched biography by Mark Bostridge (2009).

For the Sisters of Mercy, the excellent *The Crimean Journals of the Sisters of Mercy, 1854-56* edited by Maria Luddy bring all three diaries in their original form, as well as Evelyn Bolster's *The Sisters of Mercy in the Crimean War*. Occasionally I used the original, but slightly edited, first edition of *Memories of the Crimea* (1897) by Sister Mary Aloysius, where she does not use her family name of Doyle. And no story would be complete without Sue Goldie's *Florence Nightingale: Letters from the Crimea*, which gives a real insight into Nightingale's time in the Crimea (and not just copies of letters from Nightingale but also those around her).

An under-used resource for nursing history are the books on the Crimean doctors, which give more context to the medical and nursing aspects of the war. In this instance, I used the excellent two-volume books of both John Shepherd (1991) and Sir Neil Cantlie (1974) and army medical history, as well as interesting and riveting finds of contemporary medical accounts, also on www.archive.org. Whilst there are countless portraits and photographs of Florence Nightingale, we are lucky to have one accessible image of Betsy Cadwaladyr, but very unlucky at not having one single image of Mother Bridgeman. I did consult the Sisters of Mercy Archives at Dublin but they confirmed there are no known images of Mother Bridgeman in their collections. The Sister of Mercy on the cover of this book is Sister Anastasia Kelly from the Bermondsey Convent, who accompanied FN to the Crimea in 1854 (Wellcome Collection).

*Florence Nightingale's Rivals: Nursing through the Crimea*

There is one majorly over-looked event that happened shortly after Nightingale and her original entourage arrived at Scutari; the hurricane of 14 November 1854. This calamitous storm had a huge impact on the care being administered to the injured, wounded and ill soldiers, especially at Scutari hospital. Although there are many contemporary accounts of this storm, later historiographies, especially within the nursing sphere, fail to fully apply the ramifications of this disaster upon the tragedy of that winter, not only on the patients but also on the women who had gone to care for them. The storm completely destroyed the supply chain at that point, which was already failing by itself, and this event is discussed more thoroughly in Chapter Two.

Betsy's real name was Elizabeth but was known as Betsy (often spelt Betsi) in her lifetime, while she used the surname Davis when in England, as did her sister Bridget, due to the inability of the English to pronounce Welsh names! Betsy unfortunately died in poverty in London and had a pauper's grave until 2012 when luckily, a headstone was erected where she lay, initiated by Professor Donna Mead. Betsy originally hailed from North Wales and the North Wales health board was named after her.

Before taking her vows, Mother Mary Francis Bridgeman was known as Joanna Bridgeman; one of five children of a comfortably well-off family and, believe it or not, a young socialite on the social stratum not too dissimilar to a young Florence Nightingale. Under the care of her maternal aunt and namesake Joanna Reddan, she joined the Sisters of Mercy after nursing the sick poor in her community in Ireland in the 1830s. All these women put themselves through extreme hardships to go and nurse in the Crimea.

There are many women in the Crimean War that are relatively unknown and who have not only written contemporary accounts, such as Fanny Taylor and Mrs Duberly, but also those who went through hardships caring for the soldiers in the Crimea. Mary Clough (mentioned later in the book), Eliza Roberts (Nightingale's assistant) and other religious groups to name a few. There were also the Naval

*Introduction*

nurses such as Eliza McKenzie and, of course, the indomitable Mary Seacole, of whom much is written and now known about. There are, in fact, far too many women to include in this book and my intention was to focus on the relationships between the three women featured here.

From hereon I have shortened the names to FN for Florence Nightingale, Bridgeman for Mother Francis Bridgeman and Betsy for Betsy Cadwaladyr (spelling her first name as per her autobiography) to avoid repetition. Some of the quotes repeated in the book retain their original spelling and punctuation. I also keep to Dr Andrew Smith and Dr John Hall, despite them both being knighted in February 1855, thus making them 'Sirs'.

# Chapter I

# NURSING FROM ANTIQUITY TO VICTORIAN ENGLAND

*'Women have always been healers. They were the unlicenced doctors and anatomists of Western history. They were abortionists, nurses and counsellors. They were pharmacists ... midwives ... doctors without degrees, barred from books and lectures, learning from each other, and passing on experience ... They were called "wise women" by the people, witches or charlatans by the authorities.'* Witches, Midwives and Nurses, p.22.

*'Request to merchants coming with grain and other merchandise to Wenlok fair, to give liberally of their alms to the master and brethren of the monastery of Wenlok, to which lost and naked beggars are frequently admitted for their relief, the house being in great poverty.'* Calendar of Patent Rolls 1272–1281, p.114.

## Ancient Roots

Between the years c500 – c300 BCE in Ancient Greece, a new Golden Era of learning came into being, led primarily by great thinkers such as Socrates, Plato and Aristotle. In her 1985 book, *Nursing, The Finest Art*, Patricia Donohue calls them the first philosopher-scientists, seeking to explain phenomena via natural means instead of the supernatural and mythology. It was Aristotle (384 – 322 BCE) who laid the foundations for the development of medicinal thinking with his contributions to anatomy and biology. However, before even these well-known philosophers had made their mark, there was a man called Thales (c624/3 – c546 BCE) who was the first in the lands known to us as Ancient Greece, famed for using nature and environment as theory and hypotheses instead of mythology and the imaginative world of Greek gods. Thales is often considered the founder of mathematics and philosophy.[1]

Therefore, a form of rational thinking was already known in the ancient world when Hippocrates (c460 – c370 BCE) became known as the Father of Medicine and taught '… that disease was not the work of spirits, demons or deities but the result of the breaking of natural laws' and that people should seek nature and the environment to bring back balance. He also noted the importance of hygiene, diet and exercise.[2] Hippocrates also had knowledge – and taught – the importance of mind and body working together for good health (still very relevant in today's world), medical ethics, observations of the body to guide diagnosis and treatments. He also termed medical words such as *symptom, therapy* and *trauma* as well as recognising biological diseases whose names remain with us today, including *diabetes, arthritis, hysteria* and *paralysis*.[3]

Hippocrates also wrote of the physician's assistant, sometimes called attendant, when teaching his pupils and advising them on the use of these assistants. He advised that only those assistants already admitted to learning the art of medicine were to be left alone to give treatments without the physician present; laymen, however, were forbidden from overseeing any medicinal duties due to their lack of knowledge and the risk of rendering total blame on the physician. Although there are mentions of women in Hippocrates' time, mainly as wet-nurses and midwives, the word nurse – either as the noun or as the verb – appears not to be approached in any Ancient Greek writings. It must be assumed that the attendants and assistants that are mentioned would have been men.

Nursing care existed in the directions given to these assistants such as preparing poultices, bathing for cleanliness, a good diet to help with the heart and kidneys, and what we know today as urinalysis. These ancient physicians appear not to pay much attention to the assistants' lot in life and it is more than likely that the need to care for the sick in making them comfortable, making sure they were fed and watered etc., fell upon the woman of a household as well as her servants, daughters and slaves.[4]

Nursing as a role within itself is impossible to pinpoint in any origin at this time. However, by 500 BCE, the advanced thinking Ancient Greek civilisation had begun to establish a form of hospital for the injured and sick, using massage, mineral baths and therapies that were sometimes administered by a female priestess; these centres did not admit pregnant ladies or those with incurable illnesses. A thousand years later, by 500 CE, the earliest recorded mentions of female nurses had appeared. With the gift of being very wealthy women, they established centres in their own homes or had specific buildings built for care. Empress Helena (248 – 328 CE), mother of Constantine the Great, is credited with establishing the first known home for the 'aged infirm' in Rome; St Marcella, a wealthy young widow of only seven months turned her palace into a monastery and gathering centre for other women where she taught nursing skills. Sadly, St Marcella was attacked and beaten by the Visigoths after their invasion of Rome in 410 CE and died of her injuries. Inspired by Marcella, St Paula (347 – 404 CE) built hospices (resting places) for pilgrims travelling to Jerusalem and St Fabiola (d.399 CE), from an aristocratic Roman family, used her wealth after becoming a widow to build a large hospital in Rome where she engaged in caring for the sick poor herself. She moved into a hospice built by St Paula and was known as a high-ranking matron nurse. All these women converted to Christianity and used their wealthy positions to carry out their nursing. There are also some fabulous remains of a Roman hospital courtyard with adjacent hospital rooms at Housesteads Roman Fort (*Vercovium*) at Hadrian's Wall, circa 124 CE.[5]

Ancient Egypt – 3300 BCE to 525 BCE – was much advanced medically. Thanks to discoveries of ancient papyri, we know they were practising advanced surgery using instruments still around today, such as scalpels, forceps and scissors. Their knowledge of anatomy included awareness of heart disease and heart failure, dentistry and biological systems. Ancient medicinal remedies to treat dermatological conditions such as psoriasis have been isolated in modern day treatments for the same conditions. The Ancient Egyptians also had knowledge of psychiatric conditions and had a female goddess of healing, Isis. None of these historical records mentions nursing in any form, but due to their advanced medicinal knowledge, it must be assumed there was a need for a nursing service to go hand in hand with all procedures, either by men or women.

However, the Ancient Egyptian Empire began to deteriorate over many years due to variables such as climate change, social strife including civil wars and invasions, beginning in 525 BCE by the Assyrians and a final invasion by the Ancient Greeks in 332 BCE. By around the year 500 CE, many of the great medicinal learnings, writings and libraries of the Ancient Egyptians and Greeks that had been absorbed into the Roman Empire had all but been decimated with the onslaught of war, plague and the coming of Christianity. Cities fell due to invasions and people fell with them (such as St Marcella mentioned above) and Christianity preached that there was only one saviour, not many, and that illness was a representation of the suffering of Christ. Plagues such as the Antonine Plague 165 – 180 CE (possibly smallpox or measles), the Plague of Cyprian 249 – 262 CE, the Justinian Plague 541 – 549 CE, as well as malaria and respiratory conditions, decimated the western populations, while treatment was limited to what medicinal knowledge was left. Someone like Pliny the Elder (d.79 CE), although technically not a medicinal man but one who wrote extensively about plants and medicine, was fully aware too much poppy would make you drowsy, yet advised the fat of a bear and the dung of a wild boar would heal burns and scarring. In this instance, you had to hope you had something treatable![6]

However, writings of ancient medicine of the Hindu *Charaka-Samhita,* the origins of which are thought to date from 400 – 200 BCE, focuses on preventative medicine and is today the basis of Ayurveda medicine. It is within this ancient Indian chronicle we find mention of the nurse, albeit male with occasional references to females, such as massage treatments for other females.[7] In chapter nine of the *Charaka-Samhita,* we find guidance on the four necessary components of healthcare: physician, medicine, nurse and patient, and the best qualities of these four components working together '… are responsible for the complete cure of the disease'.[8] The *Charaka-Samhita* notes that nurses, also called attending staff, needed the knowledge to take care and have affection toward the patient, with knowledge of how to prepare, dispense and administer medicines, as well as knowing how to prepare healthy recipes and be pure of body and mind. Nurses with 'good conduct, hygiene, character, devotion, dexterity, compassion, and with proficiency in nursing and administering therapies should be appointed. They should be skilled in cooking soups, rice, giving baths, massage, in handling (bed-ridden) patients, and also in formulating [grinding, etc.] medicines. The staff should be willing to do all duties.'[9]

## Monastic Nursing

Gradually, after the fall of the Roman Empire from around 500 CE, in Western Europe and especially in Britain, any learning, arts, medicine, and in fact any 'intellectual activity' was centred around monastic settings. The monasteries continued providing what care they could, firstly to their inmates and people within their locality, stretching out to villages and settlements further afield as well as comfort for travellers and pilgrims. What knowledge was left from the ancient world and had been built upon was shared by the monastic infirmarian, lay healers as well as local wise women and herbalists.[10] These women, aristocratic and peasant alike, had been taught the use of medicinal herbs and first aid, passed down from generation to generation and yet, within a few hundred years, would be accused of being witches. Ironic, really, when an aristocratic lady of the house was expected to be '… amateur soldier and man-of-the-house in her husband's absence and amateur physician when no skilled doctor could be had.'[11]

The poor, sick, weak and any measure of society's *infirmus* had come to rely upon these monastic establishments for any care or shelter that could be afforded them through Christian piety and hospitality, although it must be remembered they were, first and foremost, ecclesiastical buildings and not medical. These duties, however, were secondary to one's original calling to join a holy order; the dedication to God and desire to serve life spiritually was the only reason these particular establishments grew from the earliest days in Britain. Providing shelter, comfort and care was a by-product of one's dedication to serve God and personal sanctification.[12] However, this comfort-and-care by-product born of the good intentions to serve God, gave rise to the monastic infirmary (from *infirmus,* meaning the weak/feeble/sickly). These small infirmaries developed with the monasteries and nunneries with both monks and nuns working together to tend to the sick and the poor whilst developing, studying and practicing their knowledge.[13] 'The sick-poor were believed to represent the living manifestation of Christ … the foundations for the widespread support of the poor and … the ideal of poverty.'[14]

The seventh century saw both monks and nuns serving as nurses and monastic nursing continued to grow over the next 100 years. The great monk-scholar the Venerable Bede (c672 CE – 735 CE) lauded the gifts of a particular female leader of the day, the much revered Abbess of Whitby, St Hilda (c614 – 17 November 680 CE), who was admired for her 'justice, piety, chastity and other virtues, and especially peace and charity' no matter whether people were rich or poor, and she was much sought after for advice from the common person to kings and princes of Europe.[15] In the seventh century, Whitby Abbey was described as having a building for the infirm and dying. In the twelfth century, during the English civil war known as The Anarchy, the Abbot joined the cattle belonging to the hospital to that of the convent by moving them to surrounding fields, thus saving them from destruction as the attacking forces of the Earl of Albemarle were laying waste to swathes of Yorkshire. The earl was apparently renowned for generous alms to lepers and the poor and therefore would not attack the abbey's lands.[16]

As the socio-economy of England and Wales grew and changed, so did the need for adaption to care for the sick poor; feudal law came into play after 1066 and once they were rewarded with royal grants, towns and their markets flourished, trades and crafts grew and thus the poor, the wealthy pilgrims and all manner of travellers, expanded. Secular charitable institutions grew, such as the almshouse, gradually becoming one of four main categories of hospital. The other three were leper houses, although neither almshouses or leper houses provided curative medical care as such, poor travellers and pilgrims, and the least numerous, care of the non-leperous sick poor.[17] Occasionally, we come across the mention in official documents of women in the hospitals, such as the Hospital of the Holy Innocents, just outside of Lincoln, as seen in the quotes below. It was thought to have had an original foundation pre-1094 but royal charters by Edward III state it was founded by Henry I. Known as *La Maladerie* (the sickness), it was 'intended to receive ten lepers of either sex, under the charge of a warden and two chaplains; patients might be recommended by the mayor and good men of Lincoln, and the consent of the king and the chancellor had to be obtained for their admission.'[18]

> Pardon to Margaret, late the wife of Alan Evcrard of Burgh by Weynflet, CO. Lincoln, who was condemned by the justices of the last eyre for harbouring a thief, namely Robert her son, and hanged on the gallows without Lincoln, but being cut down and removed for burial to the hospital of lepers without the south gate of Lincoln, when near the place of burial was seen to draw a breath

and revive; granted because her recovery is ascribed to a miracle, and she has lived two years and more in the said hospital.[19]

Appointment of the sheriff of Lincoln to the custody, during pleasure, of the hospital of the Holy Innocents without Lincoln, founded by former kings of England for the support of lepers; to apply the goods thereof to the maintenance of the chaplains, brethren, sisters and infirm persons now dwelling there, whom he may not remove without reference to the king, except for misconduct; nor increase their number without special mandate from the king or chancellor; but when a brother or sister dies the fact is to be notified to the chancellor, and one leper is to be appointed to fill the vacancy according to the ancient constitution; two chaplains must be always resident; the chaplains and brethren are to reside in one house, the lepers by themselves, and the sisters by themselves.[20]

Along with this socio-economic growth, there was also religious reform that affected medicinal and nursing care. A community of women were in residence within the almonry (building for giving alms to the poor) of St Albans in 1077, suggesting there may also have been nursing care.[21] However, between 1123 and 1215 ecclesiastical reform by the Catholic Church had a severe hand in reducing what healthcare was available, especially for the poor. Up until this point, the main source of any knowledge or practice had been in the monasteries and the infirmaries that had grown with them. The First Lateran council of 1123 produced the first canon to separate the religious clergy from medicine, forbidding the abbots and monks to visit the sick and perform unction – using medicinal oil/ointment. By the Fourth Lateran in 1215, the clergy were forbidden from calling themselves healers, taking money for treatments and the spilling of blood – so no anatomy or practicing the '… art of surgery, which involves cauterizing and making incisions.'[22] Men – but not women – could train as physicians, but not surgeons as that involved shedding blood, at the new institutions called universities, firstly in Europe from the late eleventh century, then at

Oxford University following its establishment in 1167 by Henry II and Cambridge University in 1208.[23]

St Leonard's Hospital in York was one of the largest medieval hospitals in the country, with its foundations allegedly beginning in 936. By tradition, King Athelstan was returning from a battle and was so impressed by the care of the poor, he granted a thrave of corn (known as St Peter's corn) for the maintenance of a small hospital called St Peter's. This gift was confirmed by William the Conqueror and the small hospital was rebuilt and a chapel and its site moved further west by his son, William Rufus. After being destroyed by fire in 1137, the hospital and church were rebuilt and renamed St Leonard's by King Stephen.[24] However, an inquisition on 15 November 1280 by a jury made up of certain knights, brethren, freemen and citizens of York – which was then confirmed in an *inspeximus* (a later charter confirming validity) in May 1336 – found that William II (Rufus) had founded the hospital of St Peter's and endowed it with the thraves of corn for the support of poor persons and that King Stephen had rebuilt and renamed it St Leonard's. Also installed by the original foundation were chaplains '... and others, and sisters, wearing the dress they now wear to celebrate divine service, tend the poor ... and support of the poor and sick there by two charters...'[25]

In 1276, a certain Sister Ann *medica* (indicating 'doctor'), mentioned in an ordinance of St Leonard's, suggests that at least one of the sisters was practising diagnosis and treatment, or at least giving care that was more than the basic care of making sure comfort was being had by the inmates, as patients were called then. By 1364, the sisters were carrying out duties such as ministering to the sick, attending to their needs, making sure they were fed, had drinks and were kept warm and to see a priest if the patient requested it. No record of actual medicinal care has been recorded at St Leonard's but the fact there is a mention of *medica* as well as an ordinance of 1364 stating that the sick were not to be released until they were better and able to work again, gives some hint that more than basic nursing care was being practised, probably based on herbal medicine as was common of the day.

The knowledge in a purpose-built hospital such as St Leonard's would have increased over the years and consisted of libraries, as well as in the monastic buildings. There would have been reference books on how to treat certain ailments and after years of practising a plethora of treatments such as poultices and wound care, a considerable – if not formidable – amount of knowledge and skills would have been available.[26]

The twelfth and thirteenth centuries saw noble and high-ranking women mentioned in the records regarding nursing care, with growth of their patronage of nursing establishments, both monastic and secular orders, driven by piety.[27] Euphemia de Walliers (d.12 April 1257) entered Wherwell Abbey as a child under her aunt, Matilda de Bailleul, Abbess of Wherwell from c.1173 to her death in 1213. Euphemia was the daughter of Margaret de Walliers, most likely a sister of Matilda and named after her maternal grandmother. They were of a noble Flanders family, with Matilda's great-uncle being Godfrey of St Omer, who, along with Hugh de Payns, founded the Knights Templar. Euphemia was duly elected Abbess of Wherwell after the death of her aunt Matilda in 1213. It was Euphemia who was responsible for the rebuilding of the certain buildings of the well-endowed Abbey, including a large new infirmary.

> She also, with maternal piety and careful forethought, built, for the use of both sick and sound, a new and large firmery away from the main buildings, and in conjunction with it a dorter and other necessary offices. Beneath the firmery she constructed a watercourse, through which a stream flowed with sufficient force to carry off all refuse that might corrupt the air ... Moreover she built there a place set apart for the refreshment of the soul, namely a chapel of the Blessed Virgin, which was erected outside the cloister behind the firmery.[28]

Eleanor de Montfort, Countess of Leicester and Pembroke, sister to Henry III and wife of Simon de Montfort, is known to have been in touch with Wherwell Abbey in 1265. Countess Eleanor also gave alms to feed the poor and had close patronage of the *maison dieu* (almshouse) at Dover, also known as St Mary's Hospital, founded for 'poor priests, pilgrims and strangers both men and women' and which place also had letters of protection for the hospital's brethren, issued in December 1221 by her brother, Henry III.[29]

An unusual example of royalty practising hands-on nursing care can be found in the early twelfth century, when the wife of Henry I, Queen Matilda and known as Good Queen Maude, founded a leper hospital in 1101 called St Giles', the patron saint of many things including those with physical disabilities, in an area outside of the City of London and, as was the norm for leper hospitals, built away from the general population. She followed the example of her parents and often washed and kissed the feet of lepers: 'Clad in hair cloth beneath her royal habit, in Lent, she trod the thresholds of the churches barefoot. Nor was she disgusted at washing the feet of the diseased; handling their ulcers dripping with corruption, and finally, pressing their hands for a long time together to her lips, and decking their table.'[30] However, by the end of the 1300s, after many years of disputes over patronage, the hospital was plagued by lack of resources and was unable to effectively maintain the master, clerk, chaplain and fourteen lepers it was supposed to have.[31]

In 1147/8, another Queen Matilda, wife of King Stephen, founded a hospital for thirteen poor persons including the master, three priests, three sisters (nuns) and six poor/infirm persons. This was known as St Katharine by the Tower as it was next to the Tower of London and is now the site known as St Katharine's Docks. By the mid-sixteenth century, before the Dissolution, there were facilities for scholars, 'a major liturgical centre, noted for its music' and in addition to its original foundation, supported an extra six clerks, a schoolmaster, six choristers and ten almswomen. According to Donohue in her book *Nursing, the Finest Art*, both these hospitals had women of noble birth nursing in the buildings, as well as within the immediate district in the homes of the poor.[32]

A Norman aristocratic widow-turned-nun, Lady Legarda, worked within a leper hospital at St Mary Magdalene in Norwich, founded c.1232 and there is some evidence she also performed hands-on nursing: '…attending upon the sick and engaged in such services lives as a beggar for the salvation of her soul.'[33]

We still have records of noble ladies practising hands-on nursing care as late as the seventeenth century. Lady Mary Rich, Countess of Warwick (1625 – 1678) was noted as a pious and able physician, nursing the sick poor in her own house with a reputation for wound care and curing disease.

> If any were sick, or tempted, or in any distress of body or mind, whither should they go but to the good Countess, whose closet or still-house was their shop for chirurgery [surgery] and physic, and herself (for she would visit the meanest of them personally) and ministers, whom she would send to them, their spiritual physicians? The poor she fed in great numbers, not only with fragments and broken meat, but with liberal provision, purposely made for them. She was a great pitier, yea, a great lover of the poor, and she built a convenient house on purpose for them, at her London seat (as they had one at Lees), to shelter them from rain and heat whilst they received their dole.[34]

Anne Howard, Countess of Arundel (1557 – 1630), established a hospital in her house and many sick poor would travel to her for help in addition to her giving alms at her gate every day: '… likewise was the reason of taking in some poor aged people to her house, and there keeping and maintaining them with all things necessary till their death.'[35]

## Medieval Hospitals

We can see from this narrative how spiritually driven both ecclesiastical and secular support for the sick poor, by Christian duty and piety, were. In the later medieval era of England alone, approximately 600 hospitals, ranging from the large St Leonard's in York to numerous smaller almshouses and anything in between, existed in caring for the lepers and sick poor.[36] Interestingly, most of these at least began as leper institutions but for the hospices, aimed at travellers and pilgrims and the almshouses, nursing care itself seems to be left to the poor women to administer. However, their reputations still had to be intact, and they had not to be afraid of intense hard work and be of 'good conversation'. A complete contrast to the standard of nurses in Nightingale's Victorian world![37]

Nursing care at this time cannot be under-estimated. In an age where little was biologically understood about disease – most thought it came from miasma (foul air) and evil spirits – even Nightingale did not initially believe in germ theory, although later came to change her mind, believing that a decent bed, board, comfort, food, and cleanliness soothed the spirit. This ideology is still a basis in modern nurse training with the famous framework of *Maslow's Hierarchy of Needs* (see Appendix 1), where the psychologist Abraham Maslow devised a ladder of the human needs, ranging from the physiological such as warmth, to food, drink and shelter as the most basic of needs. The nursing care in the medieval period would have been rudimentary but a great comfort; in the Crimean War, however, soldiers were not even getting that before the nurses began arriving.[38]

Whilst the wealthy elite were nursed and treated by physicians in their own homes, and those in poverty were lucky enough to get refuge and respite in the hospitals, there were many sick poor that did not have access to any form of care, for example peasants and those having to deal with their lot in life, such as relying on food handouts from monastic kitchens and queuing for alms at the gates of hospitals or the wealthy. Folk medicine was all they had; aeons old compositions of tradition, knowledge of healing plants and herbalism, midwifery and preparation of the dead.[39]

But what was folk medicine? Folk medicine is another term for traditional medicine, which according to the World Health Organisation (WHO)

> has a long history. It is the sum total of the knowledge, skill, and practices based on the theories, beliefs, and experiences indigenous to different cultures, whether explicable or not, used in the maintenance of health as well as in the prevention, diagnosis, improvement or treatment of physical and mental illness.[40]

Traditional medicine may also encompass incantations, or energy from crystals/rocks, but it is plant-based medicine – herbalism – that has dominated folk medicine for thousands of years.[41]

Although caring for the sick, poor and infirm became the Christian thing to do, religious fervour continued to battle against the considered superstition of folk medicine. From Anglo-Saxon amulets, magic and incantations and expert knowledge of plants to encouraging Christian prayer to counteract superstition, Christian duty was about spiritual care as opposed to cure. Yet despite this, both folk and Christian medicine survived side by side for generations and the average villager, peasant or layman would have had access to a local wise woman and folk medicine, such as was available by the fourteenth century, in most villages and homes, as well as visiting monastic physicians who, over time, became extremely competent herbalists composing many books called *pharmacopoeias* (derived from the Ancient Greek meaning the making of healing medicine). Today, medical prescribers rely heavily on the modern version called the British National Formulary, commonly known as the BNF, and is the gold standard of pharmaceuticals. One of the earliest English texts of this kind is called *Physica,* ironically, written by a woman in the twelfth century, Hildegard of Bingen, a German Benedictine Abbess who is now known as a saint with a popular following.[42]

Peasant women who helped their communities with their pains, discomforts and illnesses suffered the most over the later medieval years. In his 1992 study, *Women Healers of the Middle Ages: Selected Aspects of Their History,* Minkowski noted that although lay healers and their monastic counterparts shared medical knowledge, there were two developments that affected the female healer. Firstly, development of universities and training schools that barred women from studying medicine in England, thus creating the male exclusivity and ownership of practicing medicine. Some European institutions had a much more open policy, and an exception to the rule was Salerno Medical School, in Italy. Established in the ninth century by four doctors – a Jew, a Greek, a Saracen and a native of Salerno – the school was known for training female as well as male physicians over a long period of training, akin to today's medical training. This included three years' pre-medical study (under-graduate), four years in medicine and year spent with a reputable and licensed physician. Both men and women were therefore registered, licensed, mentored as well as offered specialist training in surgery. Illnesses such as lupus, fever, pneumonia, phthisis (tuberculosis) and psoriasis were well known, as were treatments such as using the natural sea sponge for goitre (thyroid swelling in the neck). Sea sponges contain iodine, essential in the function of thyroid and relevant hormones and, as many nurses today will know, one of the most common wound dressings for bacterial load contain iodine. From this, one can see that not a great deal has changed from over a thousand years ago.[43]

The other development noted by Minkowski was the ongoing campaign – supported by both church and secular authorities – of branding women healers as witches, leading to an unknown number of peasant women being persecuted for simply having healing knowledge. Although women from all classes in society were expected to have knowledge of medicine with home and family, they were forbidden from practising this knowledge outside of the home and for acting as a physician without the training; training they were barred from. Noble women were not always exempt from prosecution. In 1322, Jacqueline Felicie de Almania was accused by the faculty of medicine in Paris of practising without licence and acting as a learned male physician by 'visiting the sick, examining their urine and pulse, touching and palpating their bodies; contracting with the patient for her payment if she cured them; and prescribing and administering various drugs.'[44] Her skills and knowledge are seemingly not bought into question as she appears to have had a highly valued skill set and a solid record of curing, as mentioned by her witnesses. She only received payment if the treatment worked, and many people came to her when other male doctors of the time had given up treating them. Interestingly, Jacqueline was prosecuted along with three other women – Belota the Jewess, Joanna, lay sister and Margaret of Ypres – and two men. All were excommunicated and fined as well as being barred from practising outside their families. Never mind the fact Jacqueline, at least, was curing and helping.[45]

The Elizabethan Poor Law of 1601 saw an effort to bring relief to the sick poor by parish, while parishioners could be paid to nurse their neighbours as well as paying a general practitioner to treat the paupers of a parish. Occasionally, women lay healers were protected when other male physicians attempted to stop them practising. In 1581, a herbalist healer named Margaret Kennix had her case put forward by Sir Francis Walsingham, Secretary of State to Elizabeth I. He stated that 'the poore woman shoold be permitted by you quietly to practise and mynister to the curing of diseases and woundes by the means of certain Simples [herbal remedies] … to the benefit of the poorer sort and cheefly for the better maintenance of her impotent husband and charge of family who wholly depend of the exercise of her skill …'[46] These types of wise women would have been needed more than ever at this time.

The sick poor, destitute and those relying on the monastic infirmaries had been dealt a hammer blow with the Dissolution of the Monasteries instigated by Henry VIII between 1536 and 1540, when over 800 monasteries, abbeys and nunneries were destroyed and their land and wealth taken for the king and his followers. According to the

British Library, over 10,000 monks, nuns, friars etc. were displaced or executed if they defied Henry's reforms to make himself head of a new Church of England and to remove the Pope as a religious head. The *Valor Ecclesiasticus* (value of the church) represented the dissatisfaction of sovereigns and nobles going back many years of having to pay to the demands of the Pope and Rome and it was on this basis an Act was passed in January 1532 dealing with the restraint of payment to the See of Rome. Henry VIII ratified this Act in July 1533 and in November 1534, became the Head of the Church of England with all ecclesiastical revenue going to the Crown. Conveniently, this meant he could also get a divorce from his Catholic wife and marry Anne Boleyn and the actual Dissolution of the Monasteries began in 1536, creating an unprecedented Reformation.[47] This political and religious movement swept across Europe during the sixteenth century, hot on the coat-tails of the Renaissance, both of which had a negative impact on caring for the sick.[48] The full impact of these movements is too vast and digressive for this book, but to give some background to the societal changes they influenced, here is a brief description.

The Renaissance, sometimes called a Revival of Learning, was a turning point in history and renewed interest in the understanding of science, literature and the arts. It was a time of shrugging off the cloak of the religious medieval age, questioning everything and forming one's own opinion of religion, faith and a time of 'reason replace[ing] faith, morality divorced from religion, trust in self replaced trust in God'.[49] The invention of the printing press in c.1440 by Johannes Gutenberg, a German goldsmith, helped spread the ancient classics, texts and bible to the masses, seeing a return to the thinking of the Ancient Greeks and Romans. Leonardo de Vinci and his paintings such as the *Embryo in the Womb* gave rise to the knowledge of anatomy. It was a decline in the power of the church and the rise of the secular, the downside being a rise in materialistic tendencies and the wealthy flourishing under this new revival with their intellect and wealth, whilst the poor became more oppressed for being at the opposite end of the social scale – less intellect and less wealth.[50]

In 1516, Sir Thomas More (1478 – 1535), a staunch Catholic and an English lawyer, statesman and internationally renowned scholar, published a radical book called *Utopia*. The book imagined and examined a free social state on an island, including caring for the sick:

> Utopia - But in this distribution first care is taken of the sick, who are cared for in public hospitals. They have four hospitals on the edges of the city, a short distance outside the walls, each of them large enough in capacity to equal a small town; both so that no matter how great the number of patients, they aren't crowded and uncomfortable, and so that those who have this sort of disease, infection from which usually creeps from one person to another, can be moved farther away from the mass of other people. These hospitals have been so well furnished and are bursting with all the instruments of medical care, and also so gentle and solicitous the care itself, so constant the attention bestowed by the most experienced doctors, that while no one is sent there against his will, yet in the whole city almost no one who suffers from poor health would not prefer to take a bed there than to stay at home.[51]

Utopia, however, had already been a thing over a thousand years previous to More's book. Basil Caesarea, also known as St Basil the Great (c.329/330 – 379 CE) established a 'hospital-city' which became known as the *Basilias*. This hospital-city included an *orphanotrophium* building for orphaned/abandoned children; a *brephotrophium* for infant foundlings; a *gerontochium* for the elderly; a *nosocomium* house for the ailing; a *xenodochium* building for hosting strangers, as well as separate buildings for lepers and contagious diseases. Provision was made for exacerbated sickness due to the Great Famine in Asia-Minor (modern-day Turkey) in 368 CE as well as separate lodgings for nurses and physicians. Nurses here were known as *nosocomi*, derived from the Ancient

Greek as one who tends the sick. Nutting and Dock note in their *History of Nursing* that 'disease was investigated and symptoms proved', indicating a strong possibility that serious medical care was being practiced here and people were not simply just cared for with warmth and food.[52]

The second movement known as The Reformation is usually considered to have begun in 1517, when the German theologian, priest and monk Martin Luther (1483/4 – 1546) produced an academic paper entitled the *Ninety-five Theses*. Instigated by a new way of thinking developing from the Renaissance, Luther questioned the power of popes, foundations of Catholicism and promoting free will in believing in good or evil.[53] Luther and many others who were dissatisfied with the Catholic church became known as protestants (derived from the Latin/Old French *protesteri/protest*) and therefore this era is known as the birth of the protestant faith and a breakaway from the Catholic church. Ironically, Sir Thomas More, author of *Utopia*, had become Lord Chancellor of the Realm due to his quick intelligence and good standing with Henry VIII, but remained fiercely opposed to Protestantism and refused to acknowledge Henry as head of the Church of England. For this, he was executed in 1535.[54]

As we have seen, a die-hard remit of the Catholic faith viewed the sick and the poor as esteemed charity cases to be cared for as part of this faith. Where the protestant faith took hold in Europe, such as in Germany and Denmark, the charitable institutions and monastic hospitals suffered greatly when the Catholic nuns and monks were banished but no replacement was put in situ. England's sick poor endured great hardship, with the closure of so many places of refuge by Henry VIII, as discussed earlier. Therefore, anyone could care for the sick, including women of the lowest classes and also those serving time as a carer in lieu of a prison sentence! And thus began the Dark Age of Nursing, from around 1550 to 1850, when nursing conditions as well as nurses themselves were deemed the lowest of the low.[55]

Any professionalism of nursing came to a complete standstill at this point in time, even those of the religious orders that remained. Thanks to the Renaissance and Reformation, none of the intelligent, wealthy ladies would necessarily nurse in a religious setting; it was no longer a vocation of piety, it was seen as the work of a servant. After all, any wealthy woman that had to work would be frowned upon if she was not supported by a husband. Nurse-servants, as they were called, man or woman, were seen as insubordinates, drunkards and to keep themselves from falling on complete poverty, would default to hospital nursing.[56] There is an interesting account of a nurse attending to an admission at St Bartholomew's (known as St Bart's and used hereafter) in London, written in 1786 by William Nolan, an essayist writing on humanity. Nolan was present during a 'taking-in' day, where a man known as a *beadle* was responsible for clearing – moving on – beggars from the streets of London. Those who were infirm were taken to hospital and on this particular day, Nolan witnessed the beadle bring in an infirm beggar. At first, the nurse of the ward admitted an infirm beggar with decency, politeness and tenderness. Until she asked for his *wardage*. This was a fee to keep watch/guard and was customary on entering the hospital, but this particular beggar stated that he had given his last 6 pence to the *beadle*, whereupon the nurse flew into a show of angry passion with a voice that showed 'intolerance, ignorance and barbarity'. The beggar at this point was shaking with fear and stated he could not pay simply because he was unable to do so and had obviously given the last of his coin to the wrong person (who I cannot help but notice did not give it back). This had no empathic effect and the nurse was about to turn him back out on the street when Nolan shouted at her, 'Hold monster, said I, here is your wardage and may the gin you procure for it rid human nature of so great a reproach for it!' Apparently, Nolan states this particular nurse was awarded 3 shillings for every patient admitted. It is a shame he fails to state what was wrong with the beggar, but it is obvious from this snippet that nurses had a reputation for being uncaring, liked their drink, and whose first thought was of payment, not care, and, as Nolan so eloquently finishes off writing the episode with, '... shows a lamentable degeneracy of the institution'.[57]

## Victorian Britain

Recruiting nurses itself appears to have been a minefield. In their excellent 1907/12 four-volume *History of Nursing*, Dock and Nutting have a whole chapter on the so-called Dark Age of Nursing and highlight early nineteenth-century comments regarding hiring suitable nurses. These issues included women that were turned down for positions as they were of too good a standing in the community, and to be a nurse would be to lower their respect; that the nursing chores are so unpleasant it's little wonder most of them turn to drink; that finding one nurse who is not a 'confirmed drunkard' would be a bonus; the only prerequisites for employing a nurse include a good standard of morality, cleanliness, sobriety and respectability; experience not necessary and most applying for these types of jobs are uneducated.[58] However, as far back as 1793, a German doctor by the name of Dr Franz Anton Mai was already writing about occupational health, hygiene and psychology. He made a very pertinent point as to why nursing, in itself, was deteriorating and of such low esteem:

> He [Dr May] recognises the fact that they [nurses] are too often treated as slaves or as lazy day-labourers, and that such treatment must necessarily render them embittered, and claims that the best results are to be gained by arousing the interest of the nurse and engaging his or her loyal co-operation. He further gives directions to nurses for preserving their own health.[59]

Which brings us to the infamous Sarah Gamp, sometimes known as Sairy, the fictionalised character of the Dickens' novel *Martin*

*Chuzzlewit*, serialised between 1843 and 1844. Sarah Gamp has been used on many occasions to metaphorically represent the nursing standards – or rather, lack of them – of the nineteenth century. In the preface of the book, Dickens writes:

> In all my writings, I hope I have taken every available opportunity of showing the want of sanitary improvements in the neglected dwellings of the poor. Mrs. Sarah Gamp was, four-and- twenty years ago, a fair representation of the hired attendant on the poor in sickness. The Hospitals of London were, in many respects, noble Institutions, in others, very defective. I think it not the least among the instances of their mismanagement, that Mrs. Betsey Prig was a fair specimen of a Hospital Nurse; and that the Hospitals, with their means and funds, should have left it to private humanity and enterprise to enter on an attempt to improve that class of persons — since, greatly improved through the agency of good women.[60]

This confirms the ongoing lack of care as witnessed by the essayist William Nolan approximately thirty years previously. Later in the fictional tale, Dickens describes Gamp as:

> A fat old woman, this Mrs Gamp, with a husky voice and a moist eye ... she wore a very rusty black gown, rather the worse for snuff, and a shawl and bonnet to correspond ... The face of Mrs Gamp – the nose in particular – was somewhat red and swollen, and it was difficult to enjoy her society without becoming conscious of a smell of spirits.[61]

Dickens dedicated the book to his good friend, Angela Georgina Burdett-Coutts, first Baroness Burdett-Coutts (1814–1906), who was once rumoured to have been the richest heiress in the country. It was thanks to her we have the character of Gamp as Dickens wrote the character based on a description Burdett-Coutts gave him of a nurse called Miss Meredith, whom she employed to look after her own lady companion.[62] Only a couple of years later, in 1847, Burdett-Coutts and Dickens would establish a home for fallen young women, namely thieves and prostitutes, where they would learn to read, write, cook and look for work. Burdett-Coutts was also later known for her charitable works with the philanthropist Louisa Twining (of the Twining Tea family) and Florence Nightingale in poor areas of London.[63]

It is worth a mention here of Louisa Twining (1820 – 1912), a much over-looked reformer of sick poor nursing and social work. The youngest of nine children born to the head of the tea merchant Richard Twining and his wife Mary, Louisa had an older sister, Elizabeth (1805 – 1889). Elizabeth, an author and botanical illustrator, established almshouses and also St John's hospital in 1859 in Twickenham, Middlesex where she lived in the family home. This hospital survived wars and financial crisis, only to be closed by the government in 1985 to much protest. It reopened in 1995 as a mental health care facility, before finally closing its doors in 2009. One of Louisa's brothers, William Twining (1813 – 1848) was a physician who had a special interest in mental health and was instrumental in bringing ideas of clean air, education, and physical therapy protocols from Europe into English asylums. Louisa herself spear-headed a movement to realise and improve the state of sick poor nursing, mostly in workhouses, an establishment which had origins in 1388 after the Black Death. Various Poor Laws were passed over the years, but by the mid-nineteenth century these workhouses had turned into sick poor infirmaries and asylums. Louisa Twining was instrumental in bringing the dire situations of the workhouse infirmaries to the attention of the public and her well-placed colleagues.[64]

Although it is easy to assume the Victorian era of nursing consisted mainly of Sarah Gamps, it must be balanced by the conditions which these nurses had to work within. We have seen this being written about at the end of the eighteenth century by Dr May in Germany and Louisa Twining highlighted issues such as nurses having no training and being isolated from society. More often than not, nurses in the workhouse infirmaries were no more than poor inmates themselves that just so happened to be more able-bodied than those they nursed. Whilst these pauper nurses were mostly unsuitable for a caring role and often bullied the vulnerable in their care, they themselves often had zero authority with anyone and no respect from patients or house masters alike.[65] Louisa also quoted from her diary when putting across her point to committees:

> For years I visited in one of the wards, a most sad case of a bedridden and blind man about forty, who had lain there for fourteen years, and for whose comfort, and that of the kind old superior, though pauper nurse, formerly a ratepayer in the parish, who came over daily to look after him from the other part of the house, I supplied candles to relieve the dreary monotony of the long winter evenings, when she used to read to him for hours the books I lent her.[66]

Louisa had come across a pauper nurse who had never slept off the ward for nine years and was now too weak and unable to carry out the duties. On 28 February 1858, Louisa's diary noted that

> In the sick ward I visit at the West London, there is a poor girl of sixteen, a cripple, always sitting in a low chair by the fire; she was sometimes doing needlework. I asked her why she did not read, and found that she could not; so I took her a little book, and the nurse promised to teach her: she knew her letters. In a week, by my next visit, she could read a little story, and made great progress, and seemed anxious to get on.[67]

Louisa had also come across staffing rations. In the Bath workhouse infirmary, for example, there was just one day nurse with three untrained assistants for 230 sick beds, with no hot water, night nurse or call system. In nearby Bristol, however, there were two paid nurses for 132 patients. Louisa also discovered that the '… unpaid pauper had charge of the nursing in many an infirmary, and for the infirm, the sick, and the helpless imbeciles to be mixed up together was the rule rather than the exception.'[68] According to Louisa, by 1854, in London alone, workhouse infirmaries had over 50,000 inmates – to use the language of the time – seeking medical care. The nursing scenario to this was jaw-dropping: seventy paid nurses, 500 pauper nurses and assistants with half being over 50 years of age, a quarter over 60, with the others being 70 and occasionally over 80 years old. I imagine gin, the beverage seemingly quoted mostly in the time of Dickens, was a bringer of relief.[69]

One must be careful not to tar all these nurses as a Sarah Gamp, however, as that would be unfair and undermine the hardships they endured. A nurse writing in 1880 notes that

> The hours in many hospitals were, for the day nurses, from seven in the morning to eleven at night and for the night nurses, from eleven at night to five the next afternoon; and each got out once a fortnight ... What with long hours, sore drudgery, comfortless surroundings, what wonder if they fell asleep at their post or resorted to drink for consolation?

She goes onto describe some of the nurses as being 'clever, dutiful, cheerful and kind ... let no one forget these dear examples'.[70] Although no name is assigned to this article, not even in the index at the back, it is attributed to the Scottish pioneering nurse, Angelique Pringle (1846 – 1920), one of FN's most successful and highly regarded students of her nursing school and a favourite of FN herself. Miss Pringle instigated a new system of nursing at Edinburgh Infirmary, where she was a successful matron of fourteen years. At FN's request, she took over as matron at St Thomas' Hospital back in London, resigning in 1890 as a result of her converting to Catholicism (there goes that religious prejudice again). Pringle then travelled widely as a nursing advisor and remained good friends with FN until the latter's death in 1910.[71]

And then, in 1853, the Crimean War happened.

# Chapter 2

# CRIMEAN CALL TO NURSING ARMS

*'Why have we no Sisters of Charity? There are numbers of able-bodied and tender-hearted English women who would joyfully and with alacrity go out to devote themselves to nursing the sick and wounded, if they could be associated for that purpose, and placed under proper protection.' The Life of Florence Nightingale, p.148.*[1]

*'Where shall I begin, or how can I ever describe my first day in the hospital at Scutari? Vessels were arriving, and the orderlies carrying the poor fellows, who, with their wounds and frost-bites, had been tossing about on the Black Sea for two or three days, and sometimes more. Where were they to go? Not an available bed. They were laid on the floor one after another, till the beds were emptied of those dying of cholera and every other disease. Many died immediately after being brought in – their moans would pierce the heart – the taking of them in and out of the vessels must have increased their pain. The look of agony in those poor dying faces will never leave my heart.' Memories of the Crimea (1897), pp.35-6*[2]

The political machinations of the Crimean War are too vast and mostly irrelevant for this book, but why was there such an outcry from the British public about the suffering of their soldiers and why the precedent for sending nurses into a war zone?

Although the Crimean War saw the first, innovative and deliberate organisation of nurses being sent to treat soldiers in theatre, it was not completely unheard of before this; the Daughters of Charity had been with the French Army since the mid-1600s and there are records of nursing the soldiers during the English Civil War in the seventeenth century, for example. The medieval Savoy Palace, already converted as a hospital for the sick poor by Henry VII in 1505, became the first military hospital in London for troops in the Civil War in 1642. Nurses tended to be wives of serving soldiers and widows of those killed in the fighting and were therefore used to such injuries and how the army functioned; they had to be approved by two treasurers, were monitored closely for behaviour and were placed in certain wards.[3] Female nurses were employed in all the military hospitals in the Civil War and if not already a widow or wife, marriage between nurses and soldiers was forbidden, while nurses could also be fired for neglection of duties. If a nurse's husband was taken ill and admitted to the same infirmary, the nurse was dismissed until his recovery.[4]

In September 1645 the city and port of Bristol surrendered to Cromwell's Parliamentary forces and in November 1645, a letter to Parliament states that:

> … for whome according to the Generall's order, and our best judgment, we appointed an hospitall and placed therein soe many as the house could conteine, with nurses and chirurgiens [surgeons] fitting for them, and as our number increased we added house-roome and attendants to them: which though a house of great receipt yet not sufficient to hold all our foote soldyers …[5]

We have details of a Civil War nurse who was known better in the records for being a Parliamentarian spy. Elizabeth Alkin, also known as Parliament Joan (c.1600 – c.1655) volunteered as a nurse, caring for both Parliamentarians and Royalist soldiers, whilst her husband worked as one of Cromwell's spies. Elizabeth had also completed some dangerous missions for the Parliamentary generals Fairfax and Wallace and although her husband was hung in Oxford in 1649 by the Royalists, Elizabeth appears to have continued her spy work and appeared to be rather good at it. The first Anglo-Dutch War lasted from 1652 – 1654 and on 22 February 1653, Elizabeth petitioned to be a nurse for the navy: 'Petition of Elizabeth Alkin, alias [Parliament] Joane, to Council, for the place of nurse to the maimed seamen at Dover. Has been faithful and serviceable to the State upon all occasions in the late wars, in which she day and night hazarded her life, and was a great help to the imprisoned and maimed soldiers'.[6]

Cromwell had introduced a 'New Navy' with a Commission for the Sick and Wounded, concerned with those naval casualties landing on shore. Daniel Whistler (1619 – 1684) was the first recorded medical doctor to oversee this duty and despite a shortage of hospital beds for the navy, he devised an efficient system, helped enormously by Elizabeth Alkin, who oversaw the nursing service to assist him.[7] Records show she was paid expenses for nursing in Dover, Portsmouth and Harwich, although she later fell on hard times with many expenses owed to her not forthcoming. However, she was granted £10 in January 1653 'for good services to the public' and paid £13 6s 8d three months later in April 1653 for 'for care of the sick and wounded at Portsmouth, and in their passage to London'.[8] On 11 May 1654 she was paid £10 'for physic and nursing sick and wounded seamen and prisoners on her petition' and in September the same year was paid £10 'for her relief and main'[9] It seems Elizabeth appears in the records for the last time on 11 May 1655 whereby a note on her petition 'for money and relieve, pleading her services' seems to award her 20 marks.[10] Finally, an undated petition requesting burial in the cloisters of Westminster states:

To THE HONO[ble] [honourable] Governors of the Free Schoole AND ALMEShouses, WESTM[r] [Westminster]

> The humble peticion of Elizabeth Alkin. Sheweth: That your Peticioner lyeth very daingerously sick insomuch yet neither herselfe nor any about her doe imagine shee will escape ye payment of ye last debt shee oweth to Sin which is death upon this Fitt of sicknes. Shee therefore most humbly beseecheth your honours (in regard of her many former faithful services to ye Commonwealth) That you wilbee favourably pleased (out of your accustomed Clemency) and as ye last act of retalliacon, to Order that her body may be Interrd in ye Cloysters gratis, when God shall please to take her out of this transitory life.[11]

It is unknown whether her last wish was carried out or where her final resting place is. In addition to her successful spy career, where Elizabeth Alkin or Parliament Joan appear in the historiographies it is with much deference, and her inclusion in the records shows that she paid for much of her nursing career herself. In the rather limited writings about her, she is often called the Florence Nightingale of the seventeenth century and the Florence Nightingale of the Commonwealth, noticeably as the Lady with the Candle: 'The Lady with the Candle, for this heroic Cromwellian nurse passed with her candle – sometimes even that was not available – among the sadly inadequate hospitals of the Parliamentarians where Cavaliers and Roundheads were nursed by her with equal devotion and self-sacrifice.'[12]

Two hundred years after Parliament Joan, in October 1853, tensions over control of lands exploded into war between Russia and Turkey after Russia invaded the Turkish areas we now know as Romania. Britain and France, not wanting Russian expansion and hoping to strengthen the diminishing Turkish Ottoman Empire, joined the war in March 1854, with a force from Piedmont-Sardinia from January 1855, as allies of Turkey.[13] Despite the patriotic rallying call to arms and the splendid troops being marched through London in front of the cheering crowds, there lurked a background of incompetence. After forty years of peace, there were no reserve troops, just outdated equipment and too few staff: 'Before the Army sailed, the processes by which the troops were to receive food and clothing, to be maintained in health and cared for when wounded or sick, had already fallen into confusion.'[14]

Between 1853 and 1858, Dr Andrew Smith was Director General of the Army Medical Department. On 11 February 1854 he was tasked with preparation of medical staff and stores for war.

> WHEN it was determined, in 1854, that a Military Force should leave this country and proceed up the Mediterranean, to aid the Turks, should it be necessary, in resisting the advance of a Russian Army then threatening Bulgaria, I was required to immediately provide an adequate Medical Staff, and the amount of stores likely to be wanted for hospital purposes. If I had been given to understand when I received this intimation that the troops were to be employed on the duties which are usually exacted of soldiers in times of peace, I should have had no difficulty in deciding what I ought to furnish, but the having been on the contrary led to expect that they would probably soon be engaged in the field, in conflict with an enemy, caused me both much consideration and anxiety, the more especially as neither myself nor any of the officers of the Department had, from personal experience, a knowledge of all that would probably be found necessary for the wants of sick and wounded during a European war.'[15]

Despite his energies in trying to ascertain sanitary, climatic and disease knowledge from the war zone, he was largely ignored and eventually exonerated from shouts of incompetence from *The Times* newspaper (who had broken the news of the conditions of the soldiers originally) and also from Florence Nightingale.[16] Smith only had approximately twelve staff to begin with and, according to Evelyn Bolster and her history on the *Sisters of Mercy in the Crimean War*, the other two departments dealing with the health of the British Army had to recall a civilian out of retirement and depend on a 70-year-old purveyor who had only two clerks and three boy assistants within his staff.[17] In fact, not only was the unfit-for-purpose medical department affected by the 'antiquated' army, but it was also a victim of historical snobbery, placing wealth (bought officer commissions, for example) above military experience, efficacy and competency, with the needs of the wounded soldiers put second to those actively fighting.[18]

On arrival at Constantinople (modern day Istanbul) the inadequate organisation, lack of forward planning or any form of reconnaissance soon became apparent, with troops having to vie for shelter and services with the French troops who were already there and better organised. This included the French having nursing support from the nuns of the Daughters of Charity, as well as more field surgeons. Troops were moved to Varna (Bulgaria) on 9 June 1854 to relieve the Turks who were besieged by the Russians, the latter withdrawing almost immediately, and the troops awaited further orders. By the end of June, when Lord Raglan received the order to attack and destroy the large Russian fleet at Sebastopol on the Crimean Peninsula, dysentery was already rife amongst the troops and by the end of July, a cholera epidemic was in full force.[19] A British army officer, Colonel Charles Ash Windham, noted in his diary 'Varna, September 4th. — That the French and English Armies should have been here for months doing nothing, and that now, when they are out of health and spirits, and have lost in effective strength at least one-third of their force …'[20] This is corroborated by a speech in parliament by the young Colonel Dunne, hero of the Charge of the Light Brigade:

> The first subject touched upon by the Secretary at War was the accusation that the army had been unduly detained at Varna. He (Colonel Dunne) believed that the delay at Varna was the result of no policy whatever—that there was no military ground for it—and that the simple reason for the step was that the army was not prepared to go elsewhere; no means of conveyance

were provided for an advance ... there could be little doubt that the time we wasted at Varna was employed by the Russians in strengthening the fortifications, whilst our army was greatly weakened by disease during their detention at Varna.[21]

For a fleeting idea of what the woefully inadequate Army Medical Service had to cope with, the following is an extract from Dr Andrew Smith's report of 1858 detailing each Crimean regiment's health and treatment, including the shocking figures for just one regiment:

> During the service upon which the Corps had thus been employed for nearly two years, there were 1,701 cases admitted into Hospital; viz., 201 from Fever; 77 from Diseases of the Lungs; 717 from the Fluxes, and 92 from Cholera; 44 from Rheumatic Ailments; 245 from Ulcers, &c; 97 from Wounds and Mechanical Injuries; 58 from Scurvy, and the remainder from diseases of other denominations, while the deaths amounted to 112 -viz., 14 the result of Fever; two of Diseases of the Lungs; 27 of Affections of the Bowels; 58 of Cholera; two of Wounds, and nine of other diseases. And it appears that of the total deaths recorded, 80 occurred in the Regimental Hospital, and 32 in the General Hospitals and elsewhere.[22]

These figures represent just one regiment out of sixty-seven in the report, the 4th Light Dragoons. Upon embarkment to the Crimea, the regiment had a total of 299 men, with reinforcements over the two years serving in theatre taking them to 345. In addition to the 112 deaths from disease, seventy-two were invalided home to England, eleven discharged due to injuries received from wounds and eighteen incapacitated due to disease. The figures of those 'killed in action' are not given in this particular report. From 345 men, more than half, a little over 56 percent, were affected by disease or (lack of) wound care.[22] Another regiment, 1st Battalion 19th Regiment of Foot, lost ninety-two men to cholera in eight days, between 22 and 30 July 1854 in Varna.[23] Dr Douglas Reid, a 21-year-old British Assistant Surgeon, who had only qualified from Edinburgh University six months previously, described his first visit to a 'hospital' on arrival at Balaklava:

> Naturally, I expected to see a hut or building of some kind, and was much astonished when he pointed out a row of bell-tents pitched, like all the others, in the mud. I looked into some of them and found them crowded with sick, ten or twelve men in each tent ... They were lying on the bare ground wrapped in their great coats. It struck me that whatever was the matter with them they had a very poor chance of recovery.[24]

Into all this melee, came the urgent call for nurses.

William Howard Russell (1821 – 1907) was an Irish-born journalist for *The Times* and is considered the first British 'special' correspondent after travelling with the troops to a war zone; never before had the British public known the condition of soldiers during war until the Crimea War in 1854. Russell was also aware of the lack of preparation when, writing about the war in 1858, he noted that:

> With all its proud hopes, the nation at the outset was little prepared for the costs and disasters and trials of war. It fondly believed it was a military power, when in reality it only possessed invincible battalions of brave men, officered by gallant, high-spirited gentlemen who, for the most part, regarded with dislike the calling and disdained the knowledge of the mere professional soldier ... There were no reserves, no trained troops to take the place of those dauntless legions, purged in the crucible of battle, who perished in masses or in detail, and left a void which time alone can fill.[25]

It was his letter, straight from his eyewitness accounts from the battlefields and sent to *The Times*, that opened eyes and unleashed furious anger amongst the general public regarding the conditions of their troops, after initial celebrations of a military win;

> It is with feelings of surprise and anger that the public will learn that no sufficient preparations have been made for the proper care of the wounded. Not only are there no sufficient surgeons — that, it might be urged, was unavoidable; not only are there no dressers and nurses — that might be a defect of system for which no one is to blame; but what will be said when it is known that there is not even linen to make bandages for the wounded.[26]

Dressers were medical students apprenticed to qualified surgeons and, as the name suggests, were responsible for various wound dressings and some pathology (Joseph Lister began his career as a surgical dresser). Dresser volunteers were sent to the Crimea from December 1854 onwards.[27] Male orderlies were the only form of nursing staff at this point and as we will see in a later chapter, were not fit for purpose. Ironically, in the late seventeenth century, male orderlies had been bought into the army medical service to replace female nurses (also known as 'tenders'), whose tasks on regimental wards were becoming too heavy; the orderlies came from regiments or the hospital guard and would also control patients' behaviour, stop unauthorised visitors to the wards, prevent drunkenness and unauthorised absence. Everything opposite to what FN and her nurses found on arrival at Scutari in November 1854.[28]

On 20 September 1854, the Battle of Alma was fought and won by Britain and her allies, despite a plague of locusts and the cholera epidemic still haunting the troops from Varna and which took another 150 men the night before the Battle of Alma.[29] Those not affected by cholera succumbed to what Dr George Lawson, a surgeon in the Crimea, described as ' ... their constitutions had been debilitated by six months' exposure to the sun and the miasmata of an unhealthy country ... To this succeeded long marches, then the battle of the Alma, fought by men at one o'clock in the day, many of whom had not that morning breakfasted.'[30] By 4.30pm the battle was over; the Russians had lost their nerve and fled. During the fighting, the Russians had had no command of authority, with a total absence of any leader from general to colonel after Lieutenant General Kiriakov – who gave no orders and left each officer to do as he pleased – was found drunk and hiding after disappearing early in the fighting. However, it was still a bloody battle with approximately 2,000 British, 1,600 French and circa 5,000 Russians dead; it took two days for the British to collect their wounded from the battlefield.[31] The medical supplies, ambulance stretchers, carts and wagons had been left behind in Varna, along with tents and kits for the men, due to lack of transport.[32] On top of this, Lord Raglan had forbidden any hospital equipment on embarkation to the Crimea to make way for more fighting men.[33] An extract from the diary of Colonel Charles Ash Windham reads:

> On the Alma, September 21st and 22nd.— Assisted some of our own, and many Russian wounded. Much pleased at the conduct of our men towards the latter, but greatly hurt at the want of exertion and system in getting the wounded away. The whole of the 4th Division ought to have been employed, as well as others, in collecting them; whereas hundreds of men were walking about giving them bread and water, but no fatigue parties were employed to carry them in, and bury the dead, until nearly forty-eight hours after the battle. Cholera on the increase, I am sorry to say.[34]

In contrast, the French had their wounded off the battlefield by nightfall the same day, straight to their hospital tents with surgeons ready to operate.[35] And they had nurses, as noted by Special Correspondent William Howard Russell in his letters to *The Times* in September 1854:

> The worn-out pensioners who were brought as an ambulance corps are totally useless, and not only are surgeons not to be

had, but there are no dressers or nurses to carry out the surgeon's directions, and to attend on the sick during the intervals between his visits. Here the French are greatly our superiors. Their medical arrangements are extremely good, their surgeons more numerous, and they have also the help of the Sisters of Charity, who have accompanied the expedition in incredible numbers. These devoted women are excellent nurses.[36]

The Sisters of Charity, originally and sometimes still known as the Daughters of Charity, were founded in November 1633 at the Paris home of Louise de Marillac, a wealthy widow who devoted herself to care of the sick and poor. Beginning with training four women herself, they became worldwide in their successes as nurses. Some sources say Louise had been born out of wedlock, others that her mother died young, but either way, she was born into a wealthy country family in Northern France. Her father died when she was 15 and although she had been living in a convent with her aunt and then with a spinster who taught her the usual etiquettes of her social class, including herbal medicine, Louise married and had one son, before becoming a widow in 1625 after nursing her husband through illness. She had always felt a calling to serve God and met with Vincent de Paul, who had founded the first Brotherhood of Charity of his Vincentian Order in 1617 and had been organising wealthy ladies to help the poor, but the differing social classes was proving too much of a barrier. By forming the Daughters of Charity, these ladies, although devoted to God and dressed in nun's habits, did not take lifelong vows, bring dowries, answer to any bishop of any diocese, or lead cloistered lives. They served the sick poor in their communities, took an annual pledge, and had been serving the French army from 1653 onwards, taking charge of military hospitals in groups of two and four. The Daughters of Charity took charge of Polish hospitals during a plague outbreak in 1672 and took over prison nursing. They were extremely ordered, efficient and knowledgeable and, if they passed their vocational and advanced training, they were to be found on female wards in hospitals undertaking minor surgical procedures and wound care, as well as preparing and administering medicine; within twenty years the Daughters of Charity had established 200 houses and hospitals.[37] It is no surprise that they had set the nursing bar for the Crimea and were noted to be of an excellent standard. They were even mentioned by Sister Mary Aloysius on her arrival in the Crimea: 'I must now say something of the duties of these Sisters of Charity ... They visited the sick poor in their homes and brought them all the comfort they could. Their work in the hospitals is well known ... we were all deeply impressed by the fervour of these dear daughters of St. Vincent de Paul.'[38]

It is worth a moment here to explore the first nurses on the actual battlefields of Crimea – the Russian Sisters of Mercy. Although FN and her nurses had arrived at Scutari, Turkey on 4 November 1854, Russia's first organised, experimental group of women to partake in military nursing arrived in the Crimea at the end of November 1854 and began their work the next day. Despite being a lay Sisterhood, they reported only to Russia's eminent medical surgeon, Nikolay Pirogov (1810 – 1881), a gifted and fascinating surgeon who was ahead of his time. In 1847, at the Battle of Caucasus (mountain tribes rebelling against the Russian government), he was the first military surgeon to employ anaesthetic on the battlefield, using ether to calm and sedate those injured, thus enabling a rapid assessment of who was in urgent need of treatment compared to those who could wait. Between that experience and mobilising to the Crimea in 1854, he had carried out his own experiments on the use of anaesthesia and proceeded to use chloroform in the Crimea, his data proving it was not as dangerous the British – and to some extent the French – believed it to be.[39] Pirogov was not afraid to use chloroform during his time on the battlefield, and coupled with his triage system, supported by a band of military nurses and surgeons, he performed an astounding 100 amputations in a seven-hour period, apparently with a much higher success rate than the French or British. Figes notes that up to 65 per cent arm amputations and 25 per cent thigh (the most dangerous at the time) were successful compared to a one in ten survival rate of the British and French.[40] Dr John Hall, ally to Bridgeman and nemesis to FN, advised his surgeons against using chloroform with regard to bodily shock from gunshot wounds and with some of the British surgeons of the opinion it was not needed due to the 'patient bearing his suffering with heroic coolness', it is not surprising the survival rate was a lot lower for the British. It is also possible that chloroform was still considered to be flammable at this point. However, from April 1855 until the end of the war, British amputations and resections resulted in an official total of 824 and 232 deaths, respectively, with chloroform utilised more widely for this procedure; the usage of chloroform on amputations went from 60 per cent to 95 per cent during the Crimean War, although this was still less than the French and way below that of the Russians.[41]

Pirogov was also the first medical person to use the system of triage. The word is derived from old French *trier*, meaning to pick or cull and the Latin *tria*, meaning three (layers) and to separate out by examination (usually of goods, like coffee). Although many sources state triage was first used on the battlefields of the First World War, Pirogov was using triage during a siege of the naval port city of Sebastopol (also called Sevastopol) in early January 1855. In fact, Pirogov himself was building upon the tactics used by Dominique Jean Larrey (1766 – 1842), a brilliant military surgeon and Chief Surgeon to Napoleon. Larrey was also known for treating the enemy soldiers as well as his own, and was the first to assess and treat the wounded according to state of injury, not rank, as was the norm, which is what Pirogov initiated on his battlefields. The First World War instead changed the concept of military triage to include treating those with less serious injuries first, to get them back out on the battlefield quicker.[42]

Larrey has gone down in history not only for his triage method but also for inventing the flying ambulance; a two-wheeled, two-horsed vehicle that was lighter than the usual forty horse-drawn contraption that was kept at the back of the battlefield. He had noticed the usual contraption meant the wounded were exposed with no treatment for up to thirty-six hours. His new flying ambulance had a suspension system and a fold-down ramp to act as an operating table, as well as being fully stocked with medical supplies, therefore enabling rapid and immediate medical care and evacuation. After all, early medical treatment and less exposure equalled a higher survival rate. It is hard to believe that the British forces at the Crimea were so unprepared for battle when these methods had been in force for the best part of a century; as far back as the Battle of Waterloo in 1815, the Duke of Wellington witnessed Larrey's expertise on the battleground, including the efficiency of the flying ambulance, and was so impressed at his honour of treating the fallen on the battlefield himself that he ordered his men not to fire upon him.[43]

Pirogov also initiated having female nurses on the military field as they would complement his triage system. When the wounded were bought to a dressing station (hospital), the soldiers were sorted into three main groups: those who needed urgent and immediate life-saving treatment; those who were less urgent and were prepared for treatment the next day; and those who were mortally wounded and taken away for palliative care. The Russian Sisters of Mercy were the mainstays in all three groups; they dressed wounds and assisted in surgeries (mainly amputations), prepared and took care of those having the less urgent operations within the next day or so, while for those who were palliative and actively dying, the Sisters and a priest would offer comfort and consolation.[44]

Pirogov can thank his connections to Russian royalty in his venture to have female military nurses with him in the field. Grand Duchess Helena Pavlovna (1806 – 1873) was the sister-in-law to Nicholas I, Emperor of Russia. The Grand Duchess was a philanthropist and founded many charitable institutions and, much like the British reactions to their wounded soldiers dying unnecessarily, came together with Pirogov to discuss improving the care on the battlefield. With permission sought from the Emperor Nicholas – who was not keen on sending women into a war zone – he nevertheless gave his consent to the experiment of female military nurses (FN's expedition was also called an experiment) and quelled the sceptical opposition from the military. Pavlovna and Pirogov had known and respected each other since 1848 and by the autumn of 1854, Pavlovna had turned her St Petersburg palace into a medical office, receiving volunteers and donations for the Crimea. When the Crimea was finally over, the lay Sisterhood Pavlovna had founded became the beginnings of the Russian Red Cross.[45]

A speech in parliament by Sir Henry Pelham-Clinton, 5th Duke of Newcastle and the Secretary of State for War, on 12 December 1854 stated that:

> When, at the commencement of the war, the practice of the French to employ female nurses in their hospitals was spoken of, the opinion of the medical men and of the medical department was given against the employment of female nurses... The reason why, in former times, nurses were found unsuited to the care of English soldiers was, because the women selected for that service were not, as now, women of education and of pious feelings, who volunteered their services, but women hired for the service, who, both abroad and at home, grew callous, and manifested a harshness and want of sympathy with the sufferers that rendered them unfit for the due performance of their duties.[46]

Alongside the concerns of the propriety of women, it would not be the type of nursing usually experienced by these female volunteers. Attending the sick poor, maternal ministrations and anything in between was not the same as various gunshot wounds, such as conical bullet, grape shot, round shot or shell. It may be considered that the women, especially the working-class women, would have been more familiar with wounds inflicted by bayonets, knives or swords, but seeing the wounds caused from displaced skin and soft tissue, shattered bones, blood vessels and limbs torn apart by grenades and understanding damage by entry or exit wounds, would have been something shocking.[47] As it turned out, manage they did and so it was just as well that, in response to Russell's letters and the subsequent outcry, the logistics of organising, recruiting, and despatching those willing to go and nurse in a war zone, began in earnest.

## Noblesse Oblige

Those of a wealthy social standing were often expected to adhere to the ancient concept of noble obligation, i.e. to give your time, money, empathy and to practise generosity as well as social responsibility. When the Crimean call for nurses rang out as a result of Russell's reports, politicians and the general public, FN – already known in her wealthy social circles as someone who wished to pursue a nursing career – was in her first professional nursing role as Lady Superintendent at the Establishment for Gentlewomen During Temporary Illness, much to the horror of her family, and was already making arrangements to take on the role of Superintendent of Nursing (see Chapter 5). We have already seen the philanthropist Louisa Twining at work, and it was also Louisa Twining who negotiated for her friend FN to step into the role of Superintendent of Nursing at King's College hospital between Nightingale leaving her position at the Harley Street establishment and leaving for the beginning of the Crimean War in 1854.

Another such Crimea Lady Nurse was Martha Clough; the term 'lady' usually indicating someone from the upper echelons of society who was capable of authoritative administration.[48] On 2 December 1854, Clough was amongst those in the second party of nurses heading to the Crimea under the auspices of Mary Stanley and at the behest of Sidney Herbert, Secretary for War, who had requested FN head out with the first party a month earlier. Clough herself notes in one of her extant letters to a friend that she has ten other ladies, fifteen paid nurses – one of whom would have been Betsy Cadwaladyr – and fifteen Sisters of Mercy, not to mention couriers and cooks. Mother Bridgeman headed up the Sisters of Mercy in this group.

Unfortunately, not much is known about Clough's family background, but she used her society connections to go to the Crimea with the driving factor not being to immediately nurse, but to lay flowers at the grave of her 'poor dear' Lieutenant General Lauderdale Maule of the Highland Regiment and brother of Lord Panmure, who became Secretary for War in early 1855. Maule had contracted cholera and died, unmarried, in Constantinople in August 1854 and Clough noted in her letters that she '... had loved, honoured and appreciated him for nearly twenty long years! My sorrow is deep and lasting; no object can fill that void! ... I have the shawl he gave me; I shall have his picture.'[49]

Martha Clough defied the assumed role of working under FN after ending up transferring herself to the Highland Brigade's own hospital at the specific request of Brigadier General Sir Colin Campbell in February 1855, with the approval of Lord Raglan. A stern letter from FN criticising this transfer went unheeded by Clough, who, quite rightly, stated that FN had no authority over the Crimean hospitals or over her, proving that her friends were just as powerful. Clough must have been made of stern stuff as she also had a letter from Mary Stanley, to which she replied: 'I have had a reprimand from Mary Stanley for coming here; I have answered her ... one of her observations was that she thought it an "indiscreet step to come here alone," to which I replied that if I succeeded in doing good, I could see not what difference it would make ... I was in a great passion but answered her note temperately.'[50] FN also wrote of Clough's drinking habits, but this may have been exaggerated. Martha Clough went onto be the first British nurse in a Crimean frontline hospital and worked extremely hard, being lauded by those in command and soldiers alike. She had complete control over the Highland Hospital at Inkerman Heights and not a bad word was said by those she cared for. She never reached the grave of her great love, as she became ill in June 1855 and whilst an attempt was made to return home, Martha

Clough died of an epileptic fit in September whilst aboard the ship *Orinoco*, with the sketched image of Lauderdale Maule's grave in her pocket.[51] It was FN who saw to the arrangements of returning Clough's body home.

Out of the 218 women who went to the Crimea, fifty-two of these were Lady Nurses, including Nightingale and Mary Stanley. Lady Nurses were considered the only ones capable of complete organisation as they were literate and the 'Victorian class system decreed that only Ladies had the status and authority to direct working-class women'.[52] This, however, did not necessarily equate to competency. As observed by Sister Mary Aloysius Doyle, Lady Nurses had no experience of caring for a dead body and no knowledge of the demanding physicality of hands-on nursing. Doyle also noted how the four-and-a-half years of novitiate for the Sisters of Mercy led to their strength and health, enabling them to cope with the horror of nursing the soldiers; the Ladies on the other hand, sunk under the strain and, according to Doyle, 'admitted and regretted' having no knowledge of the nursing work and becoming dependent on the efficiency of the religious orders.[53] Something Doyle, her fellow Sisters of Mercy and their Mother Superior were very experienced in and very good at.

## The Sisterhoods – Sisters of Mercy

Born in Dublin in September 1778 to James and Elinor McGauley (spelling differed between McAuley and McGauley) and one of three children, Catherine McAuley became an orphan aged 20 after nursing her widowed mother through a long illness. After staying with relatives and often being separated from her siblings, in 1803, aged 25, Catherine moved in as a companion and manager of the household of the wealthy and childless Quaker couple William and Catherine Callaghan. Catherine nursed Mrs Callaghan through an illness to her death in 1818 and when William Callaghan died in 1822, Catherine

McAuley was their only heir, inheriting a fortune. It was this fortune that enabled McAuley to acquire a property on Baggott Street, Dublin in 1824, coincidentally on land owned by Nightingale's close friend, Sidney Herbert (more details of Herbert's Pembroke family estates can be seen at The National Archives Ireland), who would play a major role in organising women to nurse the Crimean soldiers in response to the outrage triggered by Russell's war correspondence. In 1827, this establishment became known as the House of Mercy, a place of safety for homeless women and a school for poor girls; this enabled McAuley to continue the work she had been doing for a number of years, including tending to the sick and needy, teaching poor children and preparing young girls for employment. The building still exists as the Mercy International Centre.[54] It is from McAuley that the philosophy of careful nursing became the framework by which the Sisters Of Mercy carried out their nursing. In 1830, the decision was made to become a religious congregation and after encouragement from the Archbishop of Dublin Daniel Murray, Catherine McAuley became Mother Superior of the Baggott Street convent in December 1831. More Sister of Mercy convents grew around Ireland in Catherine's lifetime, such as at Kinsale and Carlow, thanks to the reputation of their work with poor relief in the most desolate areas. With support from the Irish bishops and requests from the English bishops, Sister of Mercy convents were established in England by 1839 in areas like Liverpool, Bermondsey and Chelsea in London. McAuley's death in 1841 meant she never lived to see that her Sisterhoods would come to make nursing Crimean history.[55]

Altogether, twenty-four Sisters of Mercy left to nurse the soldiers in their dire situations in the Crimean War. The first six Sisters of Mercy to make their way were from Bermondsey in London, including their Mother Superior Mary Clare Moore, who had taken the habit at Baggott Street in 1832 and was at Bermondsey from its foundation in 1839. Their departure on 17 October 1854 preceded Nightingale's departure, but they were to await Nightingale in Paris, where they would be under her command due to a new scheme by the government to send an organised nursing expedition headed up by FN. Unused to such travel, with no escort to guide them and the naivety of war, the journey to Paris was troublesome and, on arrival, their original hotel had no vacancies. The gentleman that the bishop had organised to look after them had retired to bed and, as no one would disturb him, finally a porter guided them to a third hotel where they could rest. FN made appreciative contact on 22 October and a week was spent for the Sisters to be informed of their duties on arrival in the Crimea. On 24 October they continued their journey via train and steam ship, where Mother Mary Moore fell ill with severe seasickness. They arrived at the Turkish Barracks at Constantinople on 4 November 1854 and were treated with much kindness, good food and refreshing drinks.[56] The Sisters of Mercy from Ireland – three from Kinsale, including the Mother Superior Bridgeman, two from Baggott Street, two from Charleville, two from Cork and two from Carlow – were placed under the care of Bridgeman after an appointment from Dr Yore, Vicar General of the archdiocese of Dublin, in the absence of the Archbishop. Unlike Moore, who became good friends with FN, Mother Bridgeman did not.[57]

## The Anglican Sisterhood

'The interest in finding an area where ladies could develop their own abilities and escape subordination to men is especially clear in the Anglican Sisters. Most came primarily for the opportunity to do meaningful work, not for the religious life ...'[58]

Discussions of an early establishment of a lay community of women within the Church of England, who would dedicate themselves to God and serve the poor, abounded as early as 1839, but it was not until 1845 that it became a reality. The first Anglican Sisterhood began life at No.17 Park Village, near Regents Park, London inspired by Dr Pusey, an Anglican cleric who wanted to establish Catholic-style Sisterhoods to help the poor, such as those that had existed before Henry VIII's

Reformation and with adopted catholic rituals. The house at Park Village was financially supported by W.E Gladstone, who would become a four-time prime minister under Queen Victoria, together with a committee of laymen. The first women to take vows did so in private as Pusey knew the Bishop of London, Dr Blomfield, would not approve of the catholic overtures due to religious tensions at the time. The Sisters, managed by a Master, Lady Superintendent and a clergyman, would commence social work, nursing the poor at home, run Ragged Schools and help poor women. In 1848, the first Anglican Sisterhood specifically for nurse training was established at St John's House at 36 Fitzroy Square, St Pancras and founded as a 'Training Institution for Nurses for Hospitals, Families and the Poor'. This was a first for any Sisterhood as it was purely for nurse training and accepted both working-class women and ladies, the only difference being the ladies did not receive a wage as this would be seen as unacceptable within their social class. England now had its first nurse training school.

A second Anglican Sisterhood was set up in Devonport after a request by the Bishop of Exeter to help with Christian duty for '… the appalling educational, moral and spiritual destitution in the slums of Plymouth, Devonport [Plymouth Docks] and Stonehouse'[59] Although these areas are now coalesced as the city of Plymouth, in the mid-nineteenth century they were three separate towns. The bishop's call was answered by Lydia Sellon (1821 – 1876), the daughter of the wealthy naval commander William Richard Baker Smith, who had served in the Napoleonic Wars. He was to give his full moral and financial support to his daughter by signing over money to her that she would receive at his death, although Lydia was already in receipt of monies inherited from her mother. It is likely she met Dr Pusey through Mr Chambers, one of the officer friends of her father, and, along with his daughter, Catherine Chambers, Lydia moved to the Plymouth area in April 1848 and so began the Devonport Sisterhood. FN would go on to call these nursing sisters *Sellonites,* although they were not known as that officially. Six from St John's house and eight Anglican Sisters from Devonport and Park Village accompanied FN on her mission to the Crimea in October 1854. Four of the six from St John's House were, apparently, incompetent and sent home only two months after their arrival in January 1855.[60]

In a letter from FN to Dr William Bowman (who had been instrumental in setting up the St John's House for training nurses) sent in November 1854, FN noted that the 'Devonport Sisters, who ought to know what self-denial is, do nothing but complain'.[61] One has to wonder how much complaining they actually did, though. FN had followed – and been impressed by – the Devonport Sisters nursing in the cholera epidemic of 1849 in the Plymouth area. It was rated as the seventh worst area of the country that had especially suffered due to its slums, non-existent drainage, raw sewage, over-population, as well as being a large naval dock. In November 1848 a convict ship en-route to Australia had to stop at Plymouth due to a 24-year-old female dying from cholera on board, who was then buried at sea. Then in June 1849, the emigrant ship *American Eagle* was en-route to New York from Portsmouth when it had to stop in Plymouth due to a cholera outbreak, with fifty ill and six dead. Those six were also buried at sea and the rest transferred to other ships, but cholera had already broken out in a couple of nearby fishing villages. Between June and September 1849, 3,217 people had contracted cholera and by Christmas that year, 819 deaths had been recorded. As usual, the over-populated slums were hit first, but the spread was so deadly that all districts were affected, although it did not help that the authorities reused graves (who thought that was a good idea?). It was also very common, as an example, to have '… 171 people in six houses, none of which was drained, and all shared a single stand-pipe for their supply of water'. Throw into the mix the populace living amongst livestock and slaughterhouses that themselves were deemed 'revolting to the extreme'.[62]

An eye-witness account states of the Devonport Sisterhood, in August 1849:

> On learning the state of the case, Miss Sellon proceeded at once to the sad scene. In her anxiety for others, she forgot her own

illness, and finding that the disease had already made much way, returned to Devonport, provided nurses, and then, with some of the sisterhood, commenced her labour of love. It is impossible to give the faintest idea of the unselfish devotion, the unwearied labours, and the kind attentions of the Sisters of Mercy. On the plains of death they have walked, and laboured night and day. Where others feared to enter, they have boldly gone; cases at which the stoutest hearts might have failed seemed only to reawaken their energies.'[63]

It is not surprising they were more than experienced to deal with the Crimean call for nurses.

## The Great Storm

'And it is certain that a large proportion of the hardships endured by our army in the coming December and January [1854 – 1855] owed their source, after all, to the hurricane of the previous month.'[64]

There does seem to be a huge omittance in later histories at this point of an event that only added to the soldiers' plight and exacerbated the need for a more organised system of not just nursing but a complete overhaul of medical and government departments; the soldiers were suffering already before the storm hit. Some accounts called it a hurricane, whereas others call it the Great Storm of 14 November 1854, which hit ten days after the arrival of FN and her band of nurses.

There were serious concerns from the French navy regarding some turbulent and stormy weather that had been picking up pace during 10 – 11 November. It was such a concern that the chief of staff of the French navy devised a plan that would see both the French and British holding only a minimal number of warships in and around Balaklava harbour (fourteen in total to match the Russians), as well as a minimal number of supply vessels. Anything else would be sent to safer waters for the rest of the winter. On 13 November, the French chief of staff travelled to French headquarters where the plan was approved by the commander in chief of the French forces. However, it all came too late as the next morning, 14 November, the huge storm broke and the possible scenarios that had been drawn up in the French plan unfortunately became a reality.

A Russian battleship had noted in its log that by 5am there was a 'strong, turbulent wind ... rain' and by 7am it was a 'violent revolving storm ... accommodated by rain and hail'. Later that morning, the British ships all recorded wind forces of 11 (with one exception of 12) on the Beaufort wind scale indicating a storm of violent – hurricane – level.[65] Detailed contemporary accounts of the storm give a sense of hopelessness:

> But we had a sudden and rude awakening. On 14 November a violent wind arose from the south, dashing huge billows against the ... coast and sweeping the Upland ... men returning from duty in the trenches for food and repose found themselves destitute of fuel and of shelter. The hospital tents were at once carried away, along with the blankets of their sick and wounded tenants, who were thus left bare to the mercy of the storm ... At the close of the storm, the evening had bought snow ... the sick, the wounded and the weary lay down in mud. The trenches were often deep in water. The soldiers sat there, cramped, with their backs against the cold, wet earth. A still worse evil was that men seldom pulled off their wet boots ... their feet swelled in them, the circulation was impeded, and on cold nights frost-bite ensued, ending at best in mutilation ... under such diet and exposure, the numbers of the sick increased, so was more work thrown on those who remained ... the diet, so limited, almost invariably produced scurvy, and other diseases.[66]
> 
> ... there swept on the 14 of November a violent hurricane accompanied by thunder and lightning, by heavy rain, hail, and sleet, and followed, before the day ended, by driving snow ... waggons were overturned, and of those stores of food and

forage which had been brought up to camp, great quantities were destroyed or spoilt. The hospital marquees ... in spite of every effort to uphold them, were almost the first tents to fall; and thus not only men fit for duty, but the wounded, the sick, the dying, became exposed all at once to the biting cold of the blast, and deluged with rain and sleet ... Under the fall of snow which began when the storm was abating many laid themselves down without having tasted food, and some, benumbed by cold, were found dead the next morning in their tents ... The disastrous 14th of November was followed by a brief interval of fine weather ... but already the sufferings and privations which the storm had inflicted on our troops were resulting in an increase of sickness; and the horses, too, in great numbers soon died from the effect of exposure.[67]

The military doctors, in this case Dr George Lawson, also wrote of the desperate state of the men:

... all the hospital marquees [were] level with the ground and the unfortunate sick lying exposed to wind and wet. To attempt to put them up again was impossible, as the wind was so high that no one was able to keep his legs, even the horses could not hold themselves up ...camp kettles, soldiers' clothes and saddles were all to be see flying before the wind; and to complete the misery of those poor fellows who were sick ... it rained and hailed hard at intervals, the weather all the day being excessively cold ...[68]

All the medical officers agreed that sickness rates rose rapidly after the destruction and exposure to the elements that occurred on 14 November.[68] Dr John Hall noted:

These inclement conditions brought back cholera, which attacked the recruits and newly arrived Regiments, and proved very destructive. The official returns of the sick in the First Division, reported by Dr. Linton, Deputy-Surgeon of Hospitals, showed for November, 1854, a considerable increase of sickness during that month as compared with that of October, attributable, according to the reports of the different Medical Officers of the Division, partly to the great amount of duty the men had to perform, and partly to the constant exposure to wet and cold, their clothes having scarcely been dry since the 14th; the want of sufficient time and means for cooking; and, lastly, their flimsy habitations, the tents affording sufficient protection neither from wet nor cold. This increase of sickness was chiefly in bowel-complaints, cholera, diarrhoea, and dysentery; some cases of moist gangrene of the toes occurred. The first four complaints for the most part affected Regiments and drafts lately arrived in the country. The cholera was more attributable to exposure to wet and cold than to epidemic influences.[69]

There are no contemporary records of this catastrophe from Betsy or Bridgeman because they arrived in the Crimea a month later. However, there is a brief note from Sister Terrot, a Devonport Sister and part of FN's initial group: 'About ten days after we arrived, we were roused and kept awake by a most violent storm. Being in a tower, we were much exposed to its violence, and the noise was fearful, howling, whistling, and rattling. The windows in the room above us were blown in ...'[70] In the modern world, this event would be deemed an international disaster and for local hospitals, classed as a Major Event; the immense organisation needed to stop staff and facilities from being overwhelmed would be huge. In the situation in the Crimea in November 1854, it must have felt near impossible. And this is what FN and her nurses had to deal with only two weeks into their arrival.

The Great Storm sunk and wrecked twenty-one British ships, including the *Prince*, which was the biggest loss medically speaking. On board had been the winter supply of clothing for the troops: 40,000 winter uniforms including 35,700 woollen socks, over 16,000 blankets and over 2,000 capes, boots, coats and shoes, fodder for the horses, medicines and surgical instruments, as well as some 'powder, shot, shell'. An eye-witness, Colonel George Bell, who stated that the *Prince,* along with others, tried to berth in part of the harbour the day before but was declined, noted how everything, including most of the crew, was battered against the rocks. Another ship, he does not name it, saw its sailors desperately climbing the rigging for safety, only to be shot down by the Russians.[71] Although within a couple of weeks, by 1 December, there was an abundance of woollen and flannel cloth that had been made into jackets, socks, coats and stockings in the port of Balaklava, transporting it all to where it was needed was a problem. Indeed, animals such as mules and bullocks used by the Commissariat (the department responsible for organisation of transport of goods and personnel), to transport items across land were nearly all dead and the department itself was generally uncooperative to regimental requisitions.[72] An astonishing 144 of the *Prince's* 150 crew lost their lives, including Deputy Inspector-General Dr Thomas Spence, who was one of the members of the First Commission, an inspection initiated by a shocked Dr Andrew Smith to see if the newspaper reports were true. The government shortly thereafter took the First Commission – and its results – out of Smith's hands. The *Resolute* was also lost in the storm, carrying 10 million rounds of bullet ammunition. As it was becoming obvious that the British were totally unprepared for a winter in the Crimea anyway, this loss would have a huge impact on the health of the troops and, coupled with supply issues, it was a humane disaster waiting to happen. Which it did.[73]

# Chapter 3

# SISTER MARY FRANCIS BRIDGEMAN: SHORT BIOGRAPHY TO 1854

*'She [Bridgeman] had had a long experience in hospital work and possessed a skill and judgment in nursing attained by few. The hospital, from first to last, was admirably managed. The medical officers, both Dr. Hamilton and Dr. Guy, and the assistant- surgeons, fully appreciated her value, and there was a hearty co-operation between them.'* Eastern Hospitals and English Nurses[1]

Joanna Bridgeman was born into a comfortable life to St John Bridgeman and his wife Lucy Reddan in Ruan, County Clare in 1813, one of two sons and two daughters. Her mother died in childbirth in 1818 and at a mere 5 years old, she and her siblings went to stay temporarily with their maternal aunt and Joanna Bridgeman's namesake, Joanna Reddan, in Scariff. However, according to Bolster, St John Bridgeman made a 'mistaken second marriage contracted in early 1819 and made life in the old home impossible for them' and Joanna and her siblings then took up permanent residence with their maternal aunt.[2]

At this point, it is worth a brief review of the life of Bridgeman's aunt, Joanna Reddan, as she had such a profound effect on her niece. Reddan was born in 1800, so was herself a mere teenager when she became guardian of her nieces and nephews. Not only did Joanna lose her sister Lucy, but following the unexpected death of another sister, Bridget O'Dwyer, became guardian of her child also. Aged just 16, Reddan had inherited a wealthy estate and planned to devote her money to living a pious and holy life; plans that had to be put on hold when she became guardian of her nieces and nephews. To access better education for her young charges, she sold all she had in Scariff and moved them all to Limerick, a garrison town that soon horrified Reddan to the plight of mistreated and poverty-stricken young girls.

By 1826, with support from the local clergy, Reddan had built the Magdalene Asylum for girls on land attached to her own property in Limerick on Clare Street. In this asylum, Reddan and her workers taught the girls occupational trades such as laundry and needlework, although, as seen in the twentieth and twenty-first centuries, these asylums became places of human rights investigations in later years. By 1832, when there was a cholera epidemic in Limerick, Joanna Bridgeman was the belle of the ball in her wealthier social circles. However, she walked away from it all to assist her aunt in caring for the sick and dying. For the next six months, both Joannas, each with their own contingent of ladies, went into wards and schools, including the Christian Brothers schools that had been founded by Edmund Rice in 1802 and were converted to wards to support the cholera epidemic. In 1849, seventeen years after the cholera outbreak, Joanna Reddan finally achieved her desire to dedicate herself to God by becoming Sister Mary de Sales as a Sister of Mercy. Bravely taking a band of Sisters to establish a new Sisters of Mercy Convent in what was then a chaotic and socially disorganised San Francisco, California, Joanna Reddan passed away in July 1854 after catching a 'severe cold' whilst on a mission, and records show she was much lamented.[3]

We have a description of Joanna Bridgeman in 1832, around the time she left behind her social circles to join her aunt in caring for the sick during the Limerick cholera epidemic of 1832. Her lifelong friend, Dean O'Brien, noted that 'Miss Bridgeman was attractive and noble in her bearing, dignified in her address and manners.

## Sister Mary Francis Bridgeman: short biography to 1854

It was a charming sight to watch her as she passed from bed to bed with the smile of heavenly hope in her face.'[4] Bridgeman never returned to her socialite lifestyle; the cholera epidemic laid the nursing path Bridgeman would follow until her death in February 1888. It was during this 1832 epidemic that Bridgeman was noted to have developed a hot poultice to bring relief to the painful cramps associated with cholera, and she utilised this treatment when she went to the Crimea a little over twenty years later. In fact, modern studies show how the heat helps with pain, at least on a superficial level, and is akin to using a hot water bottle on a backache, for example. This treatment is known as thermotherapy, although Bridgeman probably did not realise this at the time.[5]

In 1838, the foundress of the Sisters of Mercy, Mother Superior McAuley, established a convent in Limerick after an urgent request by the bishop for the impoverished and sick. Bridgeman entered the convent almost immediately on 1 November 1838, taking the habit a month later on 4 December, being known as Sister Mary Francis from that day forward. She was supervised in her early days by McAuley herself as her aunt, Joanna Reddan, had built a bond with McAuley thanks to their shared goal to support the sick poor and education of young girls. Reddan offered her Magdalene Asylum to the new convent, but McAuley stated that although she would be happy to take up the kind offer, they first needed enough members of the community to help with visiting the sick, schooling and work in the orphanages. Meanwhile, the bishop reiterated this need by advising Reddan she could not leave her asylum at this point. For a young girl who had been planning on entering a devout life from as young as 16, first put on hold to become guardian to her nieces and nephews and now this, the orders for her to continue as she was for the time being must have been quite a blow to Joanna Reddan.[6]

Bridgeman was professed as a nun a year later on 9 December 1839 and continued nursing the sick poor at home and teaching in the poor schools. She embodied the whole philosophy of careful nursing that McAuley had originally based the founding of the Sisters of

Mercy on and took this care to the Crimea: 'Attendance on the sick is, as you are aware, part of our Institute; and sad experience among the poor has convinced us that, even with the advantage of medical attendance, many valuable lives are lost for want of careful nursing.'[7]

On 19 April 1844 a new Convent of Mercy was founded in Kinsale, County Cork. The parish priest had felt a need for a new convent in the area and was supported by the Bishop of Cork in 1841. Sister Mary Francis Bridgeman, along with Mother Mary Elizabeth Moore and five Sisters, left the Convent of Mercy at Limerick to take up their new positions in Kinsale. The young Joanna Bridgeman, who had become Sister Mary Francis, was now inducted as Mother Superior of the Kinsale Convent.[8] A year later, on 19 April 1845, Bridgeman established a new school of 700 pupils to prepare young girls for employment and who would otherwise repeat the cycle of poverty and sickness. The tragic Great Famine years of 1845 – 1847 were a testing time for Bridgeman and her nuns; a time they overcome with their careful nursing and Bridgeman's gift for administration. Bolster notes in her history of the Sisters of Mercy that Bridgeman

> … established first a dispensary and later an industrial department in connection with the Convent Schools. Her objective was to safeguard the spiritual well-being of the women and young girls of the town and at the same time to promote their temporal interests by providing them with useful employment. In this way she introduced them to several types of work, plain and ornamental, net making, hair work, muslin embroidery and point lace.[9]

Kinsale Lace become fashionable and popular and is much lauded to this day. The lacemaking benefitted some of the girls who attended the Convent Schools by paying for a new life in America. During this period, Bridgeman also set up soup kitchens and received donations from the Quakers, as well as the clergy in Rome and America. The Sisters nursed the victims of the 1849 cholera outbreak in the workhouses and fever hospitals; Kinsale Workhouse had opened in 1841 and during the famine, extra sheds were built on the grounds to house the sick poor. Nursing in such conditions, first the famine then cholera, must have been horrendous; we have quotes regarding workhouse conditions whereby '… the beds, sheets, and shirts were quite dirty and grey'[10] and 'on lifting the lid of a large cistern there were many gallons of water, my sense of smell was assailed by one of the most horrible odours I had ever encountered and I saw a large mass of thick scum floating there … offensive gases and … animal life.'[11] Bridgeman soldiered on and her skills would become useful in the Crimea. In 1861, the Sisters of Mercy were given charge of all nursing in the workhouses, giving Ireland a western-world leading healthcare structure. Kinsale Workhouse continued as the Sacred Heart Hospital run by the Sisters of Mercy, but sadly burnt down in 1922; it was then passed to the military, returning to the care of the Sisters in 1932 until 1999.[12]

We have already seen how Bridgeman's aunt, Joanna Reddan, had entered the Kinsale Convent in 1849 and had left for San Francisco in autumn 1854; it was on return from this send-off for her aunt that Bridgeman returned to the news of the Crimean War and the outpouring of the soldiers' need for nurses. We will see how Bridgeman volunteered and acted accordingly, ending up as Superior of the second group of Sisters that went out with other nurses and how, on arrival, they were initially turned away by Nightingale herself.

# Chapter 4

# BETSY CADWALADYR: SHORT BIOGRAPHY TO 1854

*'Nightingale had given instructions that no more nurses were to be sent out from Britain until she requested them. However, a second party of nurses led by Mary Stanley, of whom Betsy Cadwaladyr was one, was recruited and left London on 2 December 1854. Nightingale was not informed of this until a week before their ship arrived at Istanbul, when it was too late for them to be turned back. As a result, they found themselves unwanted, with inadequate accommodation and nothing to do. Cadwaladyr, bored and frustrated, blamed Florence Nightingale, for whom she is said to have formed a deep dislike the moment she heard her name.'* Dictionary of Welsh Biography

Elizabeth Cadwaladyr, known locally as Betsy, was born on 24 May 1789 at Pen Rhiw Farm near Bala, North Wales, and is generally thought to be one of sixteen children born to Dafydd Cadwaladyr (1752 – 1834), smallholder and Methodist preacher, and his wife, Judith Erasmus, also known as Judith Humphreys (d. February 1800), the daughter of a Montgomeryshire farmer named Humphrey Erasmus. Dafydd Cadwaladyr, a self-educated man, was a highly regarded poet and preacher.[1] A short biography on Betsy's father written in 1836, however, states Betsy was one of nine children – four boys and five girls – with all the sons predeceasing their father.

This may explain why Betsy only names sisters in her autobiography, albeit briefly.[2]

Most of the knowledge we have of Betsy comes from her autobiography, *Betsy Cadwaladyr: A Balaclava Nurse. An Autobiography of Elizabeth Davis*, assisted and written by Jane Williams (*Ysgafell* – Jane's bardic name). The first part of the autobiography reflects on her childhood and growing up but also deals with her life at sea and travelling around the world on ships; it is the recollection of her travelling that has been considered to be 'a hybrid of autobiography, biography and novel, and a hybrid of truth, half-truth, exaggeration, embellishment, fabrication and omission'.[3] Gruffydd Jones advises caution regarding the rest of the book and her Welsh biography page does state that 'it is important to bear in mind that this narrative of her life is sometimes unreliable'. This is especially relevant regarding Betsy's age, which she gave as 55 when applying to go to the Crimea, instead of 65, whereby she would have been considered too old for such an undertaking. It is, however, the only working-class memoir of nursing in the Crimea so its importance cannot be overlooked.[4] FN was dismissive of the autobiography, writing in June 1860, stating that Betsy

> … was an active, respectable, hard-working, kind-hearted old woman with a foul tongue & a cross temper. She did a great deal of good service in cooking for the Hospital. And I would gladly have kept her; notwithstanding her mischief-making … After she returned home, she fell into bad hands, published a book in two Vols: with a greater amount of lies than I could have conceived possible.[5]

What does come across reading this memoir, especially regarding the accounts of her childhood and time spent working and living with different families before she went to the Crimea, is a person who was of a strong constitution, extremely devout (she carried a copy of the Welsh bible with her all her life from when she was a child), and who was kind and honourable in her duties to others. Also, someone who was headstrong, righteous and opinionated but with a sense of right and wrong.

Betsy was always proud of her quick intellect and often found herself a victim of the school master who berated her on occasion. As a young child, Betsy was locked in the basement of her school for daring to throw the cane she was threatened with back at the school master. Betsy also recounts the time she was running up and down a steep pile of stone whilst her father planted trees on their farm; he warned her to be careful, but she ignored him and fell and broke her left arm.[6] Betsy recalls how she worshipped her mother and her memory, speaks of the love she had for her father, and how she was fond of a brother just eleven months younger than herself and her younger sisters who looked up to her but cared less for other members of her family.[7] Her eldest sister had married and moved away but it was her second eldest sister, Gwenllian, that Betsy did not get along with, stating that Gwenllian did not understand her disposition and showed her no kindness, as well as beating Betsy harshly on a regular basis. This led to Betsy deciding she could not live at the family home anymore and her running away to a neighbour at Plâs yn Drêf, the home of Reverend Mr Lloyd, her father's wealthy landlord. She states she was about 9 years old when this happened so it was probably not long after the death of her mother, when Gwenllian took on the role of family housekeeper. It was Mrs Lloyd who taught Betsy to speak English, and how to read and write, as well as the usual necessities of housework, needlework, cooking and baking. Betsy would stay with the Lloyds for approximately five years.

When she was around 14, Betsy decided to leave Plâs yn Drêf for an aunt's house in Chester; an apparently unplanned adventure. The aunt gave her money to return home to her father, but instead Betsy made for Liverpool where she had family. According to Betsy, she recognised a woman and her husband who attended the travelling sermons of Betsy's father. The woman took her in before Betsy then went to stay with a cousin. Betsy stayed with the family as a domestic worker, chasing down burglars and appearing in court against the thieves, as well as travelling widely around the world as a housekeeper/nurse for various families as the years passed.[8] In May 1816 Betsy was engaged to be married to a Captain Thomas Harris of the *Perseverance*. However, Betsy gives a rather vivid account of his demise in a shipwreck against Black Rock on the approach to Liverpool harbour on 'Sunday morning, the 14th, between two and three o'clock' and her subsequent fainting episode in a local shop when she read about the incident in a local paper.[9] However, no record appears to exist of a ship called *Perseverance* being shipwrecked in May 1816 on Black Rock, Liverpool. There was a ship called *Perseverance* that was shipwrecked off Bishop's Rock on the approach to Milford Haven, Pembrokeshire (where Captain Harris and his family were from, according to Betsy) two years earlier, on Thursday, 19 May 1814, where a captain called Harris and all his crew were saved, although the ship was totally lost: 'The Perseverance, Harris, from Bristol to Liverpool is totally lost on the South Bishop.'[10] Also: 'On Thursday night last was totally lost on the Bishops, off the port of Milford, the Perseverance, of Cardiff, Harris master, laden with rod and sheet iron, malt, and anchors, bound from Bristol to Liverpool. - Crew saved.'[11] Whilst Betsy can be forgiven for getting Tuesday, 14 May and Thursday, 19 May mixed up – she was, after all, elderly and unwell post-Crimea at the point of telling her story – two years' difference is bit of a mystery, especially when Betsy was in Paris in May 1814.[12]

She mentions other sisters throughout her autobiography: Sally, who married John Jones, a farmer; Mary, who was Mrs Nelson; Gwen (Gwenllian); Sarah; and Bridget.[13] It is Bridget we know more of as this is the connection that led in some part to Betsy volunteering as a nurse for the Crimea. Bridget Cadwaladyr, who also took the name Davis due to spending most of her life in London, was one of Betsy's younger sisters. Born sometime between 1793 and 1795, she died in March 1878, the last surviving child of Dafydd Cadwaladyr. A contemporary article states she was 85 when she died, whereas church records state she was 83.[14] As well as keeping a highly regarded lodging for a Welsh demographic in Islington 'where she was known as Mrs Bridget Davis … and many remember her respectfully, for her tender care, especially when they were young and inexperienced. She was exceptionally gifted in being able to give high principled advice. Her sincerity and virtue were part of her character.'[15] At some point, Bridget came to work for Augusta Hall, Lady Llanover, for a few years in London as a guardian (housekeeper/companion) and it was while staying at Bridget's house that Betsy came across the article by William Howard Russell regarding the battle of Alma in September 1854.

Betsy proudly mentions several times in her autobiography about her Welsh blood and would have been very aware of the social unrest in Wales, such as the Chartist Movement (1830s) and the Rebecca Riots (1830s – 1840s). These uprisings were about social injustice against poverty, taxes and landowners and were given much coverage in the papers; the government ordered an enquiry into the education of the Welsh, believing social reform was down to a good education. The report appeared in three parts: Part I surveyed Carmarthen, Glamorgan and Pembroke; Part II surveyed Brecknock, Cardigan, Radnor and Monmouth with Part III dealing with North Wales. Much anger and uproar was caused by this enquiry, which became known as *Brad y Llyfrau Gleision,* or 'the Treachery of the Blue Books' (blue books were government correspondence, reports etc).

The three authors of the report were non-Welsh speakers and their reports were deemed arrogant, with what would now be called libel against the Welsh language, nonconformity and morals. With comments such as 'ignorance prevails to a great extent amongst the poor', 'the morals of the people are lamentably defective' and 'the want of chastity is the besetting of evil in this country', is it any wonder it caused such ire? It may also help to explain Betsy's Welsh proudness and distrust of what FN represented: the English upper-classes and the British government.

Although Betsy was on her worldly travels when many of these social reforms took place, after returning from more travels in 1849, broken in heart and finances, Betsy took up nursing at Guy's Hospital in London whilst staying with Bridget. She does not elaborate on her time at Guy's, merely saying that

> Having been much accustomed to the sick, and to all sorts of casualties, I engaged myself, as a nurse, at Guy's Hospital, and continued there for some time - perhaps a year; I do not exactly remember how long. The doctors, finding me steady and sober, wanted me to become a night nurse, in the place of one who had behaved ill. This I refused, and thereupon left the hospital. I next took to nursing private patients, being recommended by surgeons and physicians to whom I was well known.[16]

In 1851, Betsy is listed on the census as a nurse and residing with Bridget. She nursed private patients until August 1851, when she went into private service in South Wales. After a serious illness and while recovering back at Bridget's house in London, she again went back to work in domestic service in March 1852 where, on greeting terms, she came to know Lord Raglan, who lived nearby; he would later recognise her when out in the Crimea. On returning to Bridget's in August 1852, Betsy continued to work as a private nurse until September 1854, when she began to read about the horrors in the Crimea.[17] Helmstadter states that Betsy worked on an accident ward, thus bringing experience to the Crimea and this would have indeed given Betsy the knowledge and hands-on nursing skills when, on her arrival in the Crimea, she had to deal with self-amputating limbs in bandages due to frost-bite and gangrene, as well as removing maggots from infested and unclean wounds.[18]

Interestingly, Betsy said in her memoir that she 'did not like nursing so well as being in service'.[19] As it turned out, Betsy ended up running one of the extra-diet kitchens and appears to have been highly valued. We will see in Chapter Six how Betsy went to the Crimea with a second group of nurses; a group that was turned away on arrival at Scutari.

# Chapter 5

# FLORENCE NIGHTINGALE: SHORT BIOGRAPHY TO 1854

*'The patient's room may always have the window open. But the passage outside the patient's room, though provided with several large windows, may never have one open. Because it is not understood that the charge of the sick-room extends to the charge of the passage. And thus, as often happens, the nurse makes it her business to turn the patient's room into a ventilating shaft for the foul air of the whole house.'* Notes on Nursing, p.36.

*'... everything which succeeds is not the production of a Scheme, of rules & Regulations made beforehand, but of a mind observing & adapting itself to wants & events ... St Vincent de Paul ... began with one Lady & four peasant girls - & no scheme at all. That was made afterwards.'* Florence Nightingale to Sidney Herbert, 6 January 1855[1]

In the first years of the Industrial Revolution in the early eighteenth century, British industry was still small scale; for example, textile workers based in small workshops or at home, known as cottage industries. Power was still driven by both water and windmills as well as horses. Steam power, canals, coal and mass-producing factories were yet to come into their own.[2]

In the 1730s, the advent of coal-powered furnaces led to huge advancements in manufacturing productivity as well as lining the financial pockets of those in the right place at the right time. One such gentleman was Peter Nightingale (1705 – 1763), who came from a humble background. His father, Thomas Nightingale (d.1734/5), was originally a farm servant who earned extra money by lead mining before befriending John Spateman, a wealthy farmer. Spateman died with no heirs and Thomas Nightingale was one of three trustees of his will. Over the next few years, Thomas both inherited and bought land and property in and around the area of Lea Wood, Derby, which had been in the Spateman family since the English Civil War. This included the old manor house of Lea Hall (not to be confused with Lea Hurst), so when Thomas Nightingale died, his son and heir, Peter, was already comfortably off. This was the start of the wealth that FN was born and raised in.

Part of Peter Nightingale's inheritance was also half of a lead smelting business. The area of Lea Wood and its environs had a long history of industry, dating back to late prehistoric and Roman-British eras. Peter Nightingale was nothing if not entrepreneurial and innovatively embraced the new coal furnaces, expanding his wealth and business, and was able to consolidate the prosperous lead melting business by buying the other half. When he died in 1763, his son and heir, also called Peter (1737 – 1803) continued to build up the family wealth and landed estates around Derby. This included Lea Hurst in 1771, originally a seventeenth-century farmhouse with a large amount of land and where his great-great niece, Florence, was staying in September and October 1854 when she was made aware of the soldiers' fate in the Crimea.

Peter Nightingale junior continued to develop agricultural land and in 1802 was instrumental in the canal network in his region; canals were relatively new and were designed as progressive, efficient transport links to ferry goods from mines and quarries. Peter died unmarried and childless in 1803 and the whole estate was entailed, meaning it could not be sold off and must be inherited by a son or, if this was not possible, by the next nearest male heir, usually a son of one's nearest descendant. In this case it was his great-nephew, the son of Mary Shore (née Evans), the daughter of Anne Nightingale, Peter's sister. Thanks to his great-uncle, Peter Nightingale, William Edward Shore (1794 – 1874) was a very wealthy young man when he came into his inheritance, taking the name Nightingale, aged 21 on 21 February 1815.

In 1818, William married Frances Smith (1789 – 1880), known as Fanny, one of five daughters of the MP William Smith (one of her sisters married John Bonham-Carter, establishing the Bonham-Carter family). William and Frances Nightingale went on a grand tour of Europe for their honeymoon, returning in 1821 to Lea Hall with two young daughters, Parthenope (1819 – 1890) and Florence (1820 – 1910), named after the cities they were born in during their travels. On their return to England, the family stayed at Lea Hall, which was not to Fanny's liking, so Lea Hurst was rebuilt and enlarged to be a comfortable fifteen-bedroom country home, completed in 1823. The Nightingales relocated to somewhere more socially connected and moved to the Embley estate in Hampshire in 1826, becoming the neighbour of Lord Palmerston, who would later play a pivotal role in the Crimea. The Nightingales' Derbyshire home was used as a country retreat thereafter.[3]

According to her 2009 biographer, Bostridge notes that FN had a rather sickly childhood and appeared to have trouble adjusting to the dampness of the English climate after spending her first year of life in warmer European climates, suffering from illness such as coughs, constant sore throats and trouble with her wrist and ankle joints.[4] She was writing from a young age, her earliest surviving letter dates from 1827 and she could speak and write fluent French by the time she was nine. During childhood games, she would like to be the leader amongst her cousins and her older sister, Parthenope, remembers her as wildly spirited, fun and extremely enquiring of everything. By 1831, she had become 'increasingly morose and withdrawn' and this inward reflection was noted by family members as a cause for concern. That same year, her father took over the academic teaching of his daughters and FN rose to the occasion, whereas her sister admitted that she was not as strict or focused as FN. By her late teens, FN was fluent in French, Italian, Latin and Greek and later knew Hebrew and German. She flourished in learning maths, history, chemistry, geography, physics, astronomy, philosophy, grammar and composition, and the survival of her many letters today show how fond she was of writing, albeit with occasional exaggerated flourishes of the English language.[6]

It has been widely written the FN suffered bouts of depression, illness and unworthiness in her role in life; unlike her sister who was happy to live the life of a wealthy young lady to whom marriage was the ultimate goal. FN often pondered what her role was in life through a lot of self-examination, something she had done as a young child; even at that young age, she was always with her mother on charity works including supporting a poor school and visiting poor neighbours.[7] As she got older, it was FN who cared and nursed for others in the family when they were ill and who helped nurse the sick poor in the local village of Wellow, next to her family estate in Embley, Hampshire. It was at Embley, on 7 February 1837, aged just 17, FN felt she had a calling from God to serve and although unsure where or how, she felt it was to serve the poor and do charitable works; she had been nursing family and friends through an influenza outbreak when this epiphany happened. After another family trip abroad shortly after this revelation, in the summer of 1845, FN once again became heavily involved in nursing in the local village but was becoming frustrated at her lack of knowledge and of those around her; in her 1931 biography of FN, O'Malley states:

> This lack of training among those who ministered to the sick was general. She saw a woman poisoned by the fools who were looking after her as truly as if they had given her arsenic. She saw all round her suffering which might have been prevented or at least alleviated, if only those in attendance had known what to do and how to do it.[7]

It was around this time FN formed a plan; Dr Fowler, a friend of the Nightingales, had been a physician at Salisbury Infirmary and he and his wife were coming to stay with them that Christmas. FN liked the way he thought and how he embraced changes that happened in the medical world. Being a dutiful daughter, she realised her mother would not be able to spare her from the family estates for long, but formed a plan to train at Salisbury Infirmary for about three months and then set up a small nursing facility in her local village. In a letter to a cousin in December 1845, FN wrote about plans to set up something akin to a Protestant Sisterhood, without vows, in her local village after having some hospital training.[8]

It is well known that FN's family were not happy about her wish to nurse in one form or another, as well as her hesitance of falling into the expectation of marrying and having children, as was expected of someone within her social milieu. Her mother strictly forbade such an endeavour as Salisbury and was horrified to say the least: 'She might encounter patients suffering from diseases a lady could not even think of, and certainly could not mention. Worst of all, she might be exposed to vulgar advances from surgeons who were not gentlemen.'[9] One can only imagine FN's despondency. At that point, Selina and Charles Bracebridge, who met the Nightingales on previous travels abroad, convinced her parents that she should travel to Rome with them for the winter, with Selina Bracebridge perceptive to FN's need to do something outside of her social standing. Her parents, worried about her health at this time, agreed.

It was during this trip that FN met Sidney Herbert and his wife Mary, as well as Dr Henry Manning and Mary Stanley, all of whom would play a critical part in her Crimean experience. She also met and spent a lot of time with the Roman Catholic nun, Laura de Saint Colombe, also known as Madre Colomba, of the convent Trinità dei Monti, who became her spiritual mentor whilst FN experienced a ten-day retreat there. It was during this time that FN dabbled with converting to Catholicism, primarily for its enablement for women independent from the outside world, but decided against joining as she felt her calling was to actually be part of the world, especially nursing the sick. Madre Colomba, however, encouraged FN's calling and took FN's visions of holy messages, to work with God, very seriously and was her most ardent supporter at this time.

When FN returned to Embley from this trip, she spent much time working with poor children and the Ragged Schools both locally and in Westminster. In October/November 1849 she again joined the Bracebridges on their travels to Egypt, much to the delight of her parents and sister who now hoped FN would become a woman of scholarly and literary passions. The journey home via Germany would mark the biggest turning point in FN's life so far; with a degree of support from Selina Bracebridge, FN spent two weeks at the Deaconess Institute at Kaiserswerth.[10]

Kaiserswerth, a town on the river Rhine, in Dusseldorf, North Germany had a long history, having had a Benedictine Abbey built there around the year 700 CE. Over a thousand years later, it was mainly known for its support of female prisoners and then its training of nurses. A deacon, derived from the Ancient Greek word *diakonos* meaning helper/servant, was part of a church ministry and as we saw in Chapter One, was used for the females who nursed other females and the poor. A deaconess, therefore, became an ancient order of nurses and although the role was abolished from the church c.533 CE, deaconesses were revived by the protestant church in the nineteenth century and in 1836, Pastor Theodor Fliedner and his first wife Friederike, established what would become a major regenerating movement of nurse training – the Deaconess Institute of Kaiserswerth. What started as a small refuge in a cottage for discharged women prisoners became a large Protestant Motherhouse, not dependent on the church and no rule to take vows. The deaconesses were unpaid, but that was the point of a Motherhouse, where they lived free in return for their work. There were two work streams at Kaiserswerth: Nursing and Poor Relief. Nursing entailed hospital, private and parish/district nursing; Poor Relief covered almshouses, asylums, training homes for servants, orphanages and homes for the aged and infirm. By the early twentieth century, the Kaiserwerth Institute was capable of training up to 4,000 women.[11]

FN arrived at Kaiserwerth on 31 July 1850 and stayed for two weeks, studying and observing the work of the Pastor and his second wife, Caroline. According to FN's diary, she left Kaiserswerth on 13 August and rejoined the Bracebridges in Dusseldorf. They then stayed at Ghent while FN continued writing her pamphlet, which was completed and sent off by Mr Bracebridge by 19 August and the party returned to England shortly after. The pamphlet, with the rather long title of *The Institution of Kaiserswerth on the Rhine, for the Practical Training of Deaconesses, under the direction of the Rev. Pastor Fliedner, embracing the Support and Care of a Hospital, Infant and Industrial schools, and a Female Penitentiary* was published anonymously in 1851, although this was FN's first published paper.[12]

> Another secret of Pastor Fliedner's education is, that he really, not nominally, delegates his authority. Every master and parent knows how difficult this is. He does not like to see another do ill, what he can do well. He doubts how far it is right to allow it, and much as he feels the importance of forming his monitors or children, he ends by waiting till they are fit for their office ... Pastor Fliedner ... guards both them [nurses] and the patients from danger. Every week he gives a lecture to the nurses, before which, each has to report to him all that she has read to her patients ... and receive his advice as to how she should proceed.[13]

Was this the foundation of FN's management of her nurses in the Crimea? She returned for a three-month stay at Kaiserwerth a year later, from July to October 1851, where she practised clinical nursing including assisting during an amputation.[14] In February 1853 she spent time observing the hospitals of Paris and staying with the Sisters of Charity and working in their hospital for a short period. These years trying to find her direction were played against the background of FN's family's distress at her choice of life; her mother lamented the waste of intelligence in her daughter, whilst her sister suffered something akin to a nervous breakdown. FN's father eventually broke the stalemate, after much input from their respected friends such as the Bracebridges and Herberts, who supported FN, by giving his daughter a yearly allowance of £500, approximately £50,000 in today's money [Bank of England calculator]. She now had her freedom.[15]

As we have seen, when the Crimean call for nurses rang out, FN was in her first professional nursing role as Lady Superintendent at the Establishment for Gentlewomen During Temporary Illness. This six-bed establishment had been founded in 1849 by Lady Charlotte Canning, wife of Sir Charles Canning and a favourite lady in waiting of Queen Victoria; she was also a contemporary of FN. The house, then at No.8 Chandos Street, Cavendish Square, London, opened its doors on 15 March 1850 to women who were wealthy enough to pay to stay for medical care, but not wealthy enough to have privately attending doctors or nurses; due to class values in Victorian England, it would also be looked upon as unseemly if they attended a public hospital. The Establishment had run into difficulties by winter 1853, when FN was then approached, after the committee had had problems with retaining an efficient nursing staff, often using nurses from Elizabeth Fry's institution.

Elizabeth Fry, née Gurney (1780 – 1845), was born into a wealthy Norfolk Quaker family, being the fourth of twelve children – seven daughters and five sons – and married a fellow Quaker, the wealthy Joseph Fry in 1800, having eleven children of her own. More known for her work on prison reform for inmates and their children, but less known in nursing history, Elizabeth was apparently dyslexic and not as a quick learner as her siblings, so her family considered her not worthy of a good education. Elizabeth, however, was actually a very active philanthropist, establishing libraries for the coastguard and navy as well as saving societies for the poor. She would go onto to establish the country's first secular nursing school, known as the

Institute of Nursing Sisters, in London, in 1840 with the help of Dowager Queen Adelaide and the Bishop of London, at some attempt to regulate women who nursed the sick poor. It was borne on the foundation to '... provide experienced, conscientious and Christian nurses for the sick, and also to raise the standard of this useful and important occupation ... suitable women are selected with great care, and their characters minutely enquired to.' Although the Institute had overtones of a Sisterhood, this protestant but secular nursing school, firstly in Whitechapel and then Devonshire Square, had nurses that were utilised by both Guy's and St Thomas' in London. By 1848, this Institute of Nursing Sisters was setting a precedent in carving a successful pathway to deliver a form of nurse training to make the profession respectable.

Praised by the male doctors, who called Fry the founder of nursing, and noted as 'the real pioneer of nursing' by the nurse historian Margaret Breay (1862 – 1939), FN was a donator to the Institution and approached them in her initial plans to go to the Crimea. However, the governors wanted to retain control of their nurses, which FN was unable to do due to having to report to the War Office, the military officers and army doctors, so Fry's nurses were actually absent from the original nursing party; they did eventually send three nurses to the army and three to the naval hospitals.[16]

Originally there had been a matron, a cook, a kitchen and house maid, and a manservant, as well as doctors and surgeons who gave their time voluntarily to the Establishment for Gentlewomen During Temporary Illness. One of these doctors was Dr Henry Bence Jones, an accomplished physician at St George's hospital who also studied chemistry in relation to health and disease, earning the plaudit of 'being the best chemical doctor in London'. He also developed the Bence-Jones test for detecting protein in urine, possibly indicating forms of myeloma and still in use today. He was the personal physician of Sidney Herbert – he and Herbert had attended Harrow School together. Bence Jones (he never hyphenated his surname in his own lifetime) and Herbert were also on the council elected by

FN whilst still in the Crimea that managed The Nightingale Fund, which was set up in England after FN had recovered from a serious illness in the Crimea as a way to express people's gratitude for the work she was doing. Bence Jones was also interested in setting up a nurse training school in his hospital, St George's, and asked FN on her return for her help, but although FN refused, she was gratefully aware of his support for nursing education and improvements of sanitation, despite the fact they often disagreed on many things. The Nightingale Fund ended up being the foundation of FN's training school at St Thomas'.[17]

Originally, matrons headed up what nursing there was from when the Establishment for Gentlewomen During Temporary Illness first opened. The first, Miss Hall, started in March 1850 and was dismissed a few days later; her successor, Miss Woolley, had been dismissed by October 1851 and at the end of that year, the committee changed the policy of the House and redefined the roles of the cook and maids. The biggest change was that of Matron to Lady Superintendent, to cover nursing as well as the administration and management of the place.[18] Their first choice, a Mrs Helps (no pun intended!) declined the offer and there followed a period of no Matron/Superintendent before a temporary lady who was also dismissed due to her 'disreputable behaviour'. The term 'Lady Superintendent' was used to distinguish the Lady from the lower working-class 'Matron' and FN ticked all their boxes due to her social milieu, and her experiences at Kaiserswerth and Paris.

In February 1853, FN laid out her requirements if she was to accept the post; this included employing and discharging nurses without committee interference, the reorganisation of the establishment and introducing a training school for nursing. She also requested to manage the budget, choose a chaplain and new premises. This was agreed and FN formerly accepted the position on 28 April 1853. In June of that year, the Establishment found new premises in the developing area of Harley Street, named after the 2nd Earl of Oxford, Edward Harley, whose marriage in 1713 had bought him the land

and environs of the then-villages of Marylebone and Tyburn. By 1860, the developing area had attracted the likes of military men and scientists, with the medical fraternity using the spacious houses for both residence and surgery. Lady Canning's foundation had therefore been very forward thinking.[19]

FN took up residency on 12 August 1853 at No.1 Upper Harley Street and wrote the first of her quarterly reports to the committee on 14 November 1853. As well as spending details, she remarks on the 'most dirty and neglected' state of the linen and furniture on moving from the old to the new Institution. She changed the household staff by reducing to one, as well as the nurses, except for one called Nurse Smith, but goes on to state she is satisfied with three nurses, one on each floor. She changed the duties of bread-making and preserving to be done in the home itself to save money and had prepared the accommodation for twenty-seven patients. During this quarter, FN states she had eighteen patients with thirteen still left at the time of writing, while five were discharged: one wishing to return home as suffering with an 'internal incurable tumour'; one benefitting from Amaurosis (temporary blindness in one eye); one cured by an operation to remove a 'cancer of the breast'; one cured from 'weakness' by leaving for New Zealand and finally, one discharged due to being inappropriate for the Institution – she had chronic rheumatism.[20] In fact, by the December, FN had noticed over time that genuine hospital cases for this particular Institution were being overtaken by the more enduring chronic illnesses and those that were admitted by families as an asylum.

In her quarterly report of February 1854, Nightingale made five specific requests of the committee to a) limit admissions to cases of serious illness only; b) any others were on approval for a week or two only when they should then depart 'if the Medical Officers declare them unlikely to benefit by medical treatment'; c) to reinforce the rule that the stay of the patient be limited to two months (as was the rule in the hospitals generally) unless recovery or death is expected on opinion, again, of the Medical Officers. The last two, D and E, are what we today would recognise as social needs; d) FN suggested that Lady Visitors could assist the medical men in 'turning the patients out of themselves and their comforts' and to e) encourage efforts of those patients discharged to find occupations. Nightingale concluded that patients were more interested in eating and (specifically) drinking and stated that if not enforced, the Institution would become 'not a Hospital for the Sick, but a Hospital for incompatible tempers and for hysterical fancies'.[21]

FN specified that her Harley Street contract would end if she had not initiated her planned nurse training school after a year in post. In her quarterly report on 7 August 1854, she noted that, 'I have not effected anything towards the object of training nurses ... in every other respect, viz, as to good order, good nursing, moral influence & economy, the result has been to me most satisfactory.'[22] In fact, two months earlier, in July 1854, King's College Hospital had already approached Nightingale and negotiations were underway for her to set up a nurse training school, although the talks were hush-hush.[23] This is the situation FN was in when the advent of the Crimea War changed her path. But what became of the Harley Street clinic she had been the head of for a year? Indeed, it is still standing today as a private mental health facility. In 1866, the address went from No.1 to No. 90 Harley Street due to the geographical unifying of Upper and Lower Harley Street but by 1900, the institution was struggling financially. The lease was due to expire in 1909 and a new plot of land nearby, Lisson Grove, was purchased and a new nursing home built with thirty-two beds, which was opened on 7 March 1910 by the Princess of Wales, later Queen Mary. When FN died on 13 August the same year, the building was renamed the Florence Nightingale Hospital for Gentlewomen and was extended in 1912 to accommodate an extra six beds before being officially opened on 14 November 1913 by the Duchess of Albany. It became part of the Second World War effort (Emergency Medical Service) with thirty-eight beds and was exempt from the launch of the National Health Service in 1948, remaining a private and independent hospital. In 1978 it came under the auspices of BUPA and by 2010 was specialising in psychological issues, addictions and eating disorders by a private health care company and today remains a private mental health hospital called The Nightingale Hospital, still based in Lisson Grove.[24]

Whilst at Harley Street, at the end of August 1854, an outbreak of cholera in and around Soho saw FN volunteer her services at the Middlesex Hospital. When the worst was over, FN took a short break to recover at the family home of Lea Hurst. After reading the same reports coming from the Crimea as everyone else, she left Lea Hurst on 10 October to return to London, where she wasted no time in planning to help answer the desperate call for nurses.[25] Strangely, her original biographer, Cook, does not mention any of this, only from when FN had privately sorted a small party and wrote to Sidney Herbert.

By 14 October 1854, Nightingale had already been making private arrangements to take a small nursing party to the Crimea, with or without government assistance. By 11 October, Lady Maria Forester (d. March 1894), daughter of 3rd Earl of Roden and widow of the Honourable Charles Forester (d.1852) had already discussed financing three nurses, at a cost of £200 (approximately £17,500 today) to go to the Crimea with FN, who would take one of her own nurses with her. Lady Forester had already gained personal – but unofficial – permission from Lord Palmerston, as well as an agreement with Dr Andrew Smith, the head of the Army Medical Department, who had promised to supply FN with letters to Dr Menzies, the chief medical officer at Scutari. Smith also reassured FN that she would find all working well at Scutari and he approved of females going into the military hospitals for their skills at support and comfort. The meeting was brief but would come back to haunt Smith a mere three months later.[26] Lady Forester admitted she would be 'useless' trying to lead nurses in a military hospital but was a fine example of the Victorian upper class using her societal connections as well as her noblesse oblige.

In her letter dated 14 October, FN wrote to her good friend Elizabeth Herbert, wife of the Secretary at War, Sidney Herbert, all well associated in their social circles.[27] In her letter, she was asking for guidance on procedures and protocols for her planned expedition, as well as a leave of absence from her role as Superintendent at the Harley Street Clinic:

> A small private expedition of nurses has been organized for Scutari, and I have been asked to command it. I take myself out and one nurse ... Lady Maria Forester has given £200 to take out three others. We feed and lodge ourselves there and are to be no expense whatever to the country. Lord Clarendon (Foreign Secretary) has been asked by Lord Palmerston (Home Secretary) to write to Lord Stratford (Ambassador to Constantinople) for us, and has consented ... Unless my Ladies' Committee feel that this is a thing which appeals to the sympathies of all, and urge me, rather than barely consent, I cannot honourably break my engagement here. And I write to you as one of my mistresses ... What does Mr. Herbert say to the scheme itself? Does he think it will be objected to by the authorities? Would he give us any advice or letters of recommendation?[28]

By coincidence, Sidney Herbert was ahead of FN and sent a letter to her on 15 October requesting she head up an official nursing expedition to the Crimean War. Unfortunately, however, it crossed with FN's:

> It would be impossible to carry about a large staff of female nurses with the army in the field. But at Scutari, having now a fixed hospital, no military reason exists against their introduction, and I am confident they might be introduced with great benefit, for hospital orderlies must be very rough hands, and most of them, on such an occasion as this, very inexperienced ones ... There is but one person in England that I know of who would

be capable of organizing and superintending such a scheme; and I have been several times on the point of asking you hypothetically if, supposing the attempt were made, you would undertake to direct it.[29]

On 16 October, Herbert and FN met in person and on the 18th, Herbert presented the plan to the government for FN to head up an organised nursing party. It received unanimous support, with the Admiralty ordered to provide the passage to Constantinople for the party. Three days later, FN left London for Scutari with her band of selected nurses.[30]

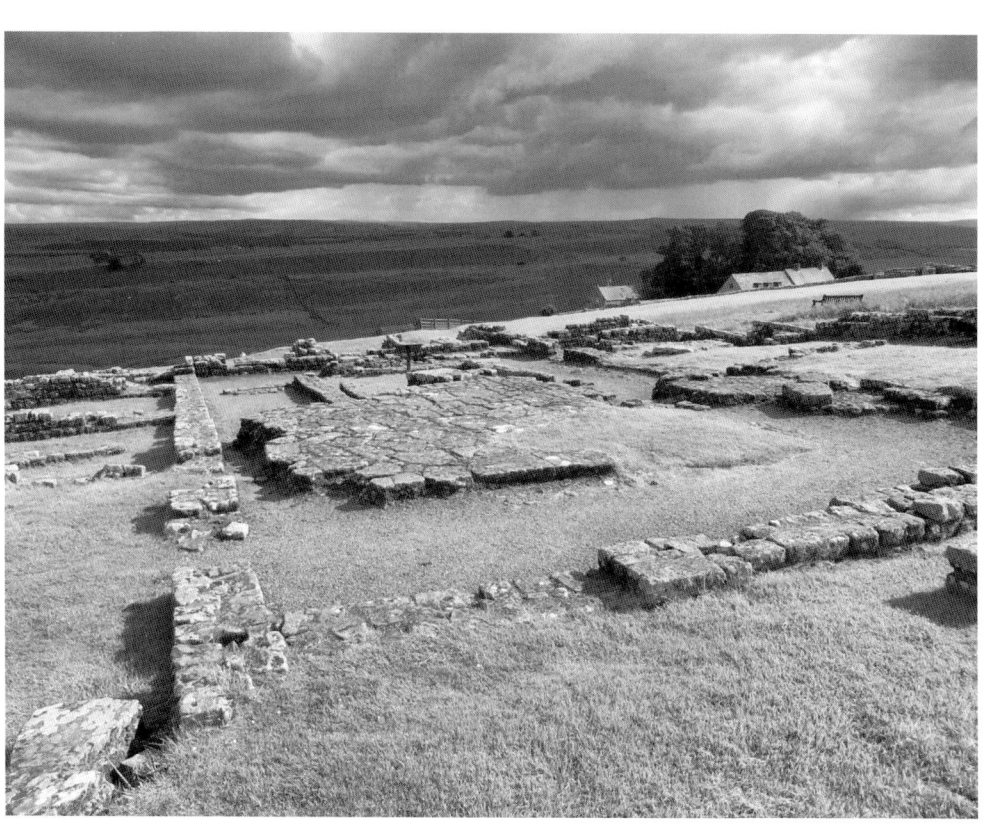

Hospital building at Housesteads Roman Fort, Hadrian's Wall. An expanse of the paved floor of the hospital courtyard can be seen in the centre of the photograph. Rooms would have opened on to it from all four sides. (Duncan Graham CC BY-SA 2.09 at geograph.co.uk)

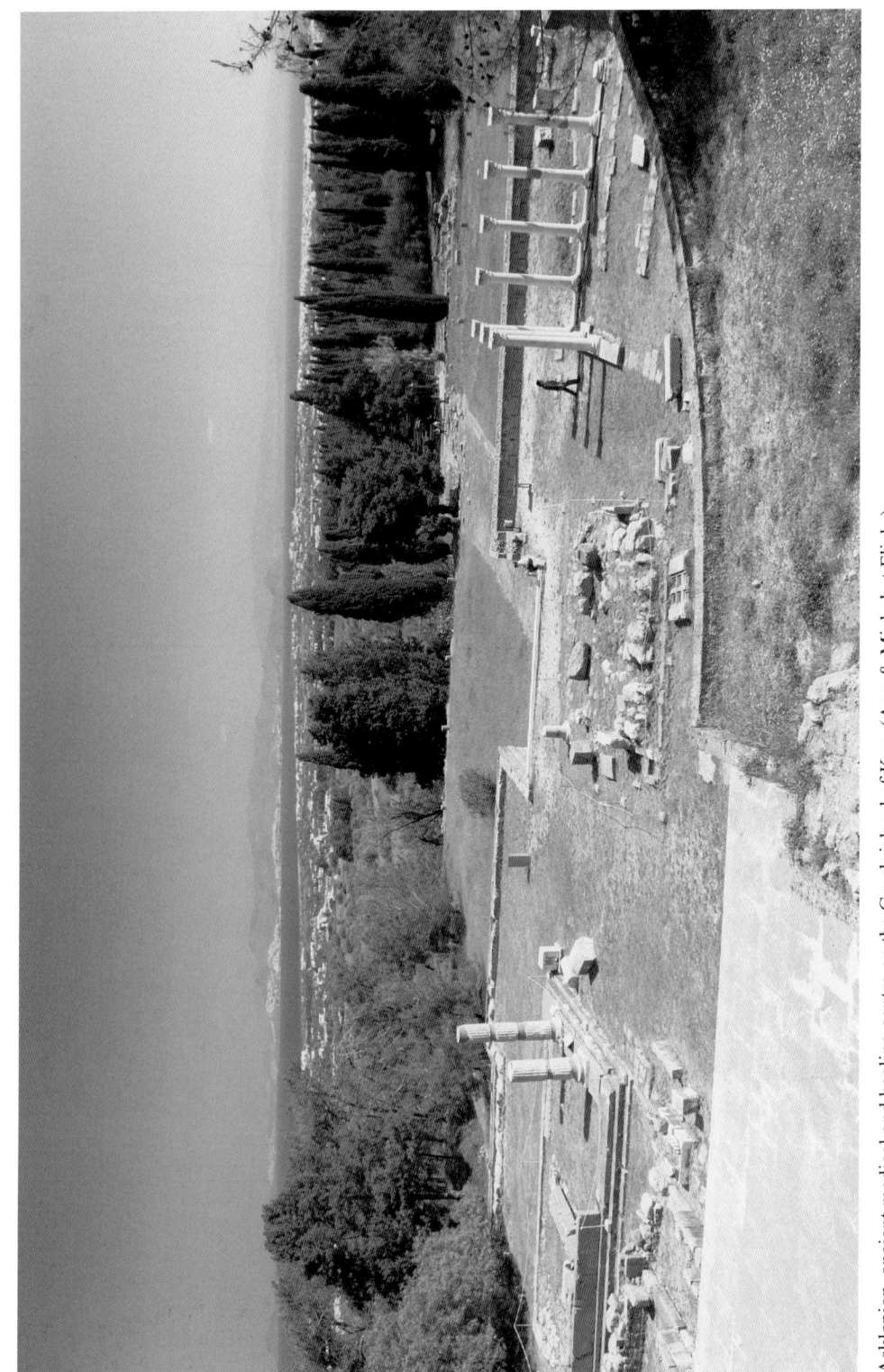

Asklepion, ancient medical and healing centre on the Greek island of Kos. (Ann & Michal at Flickr)

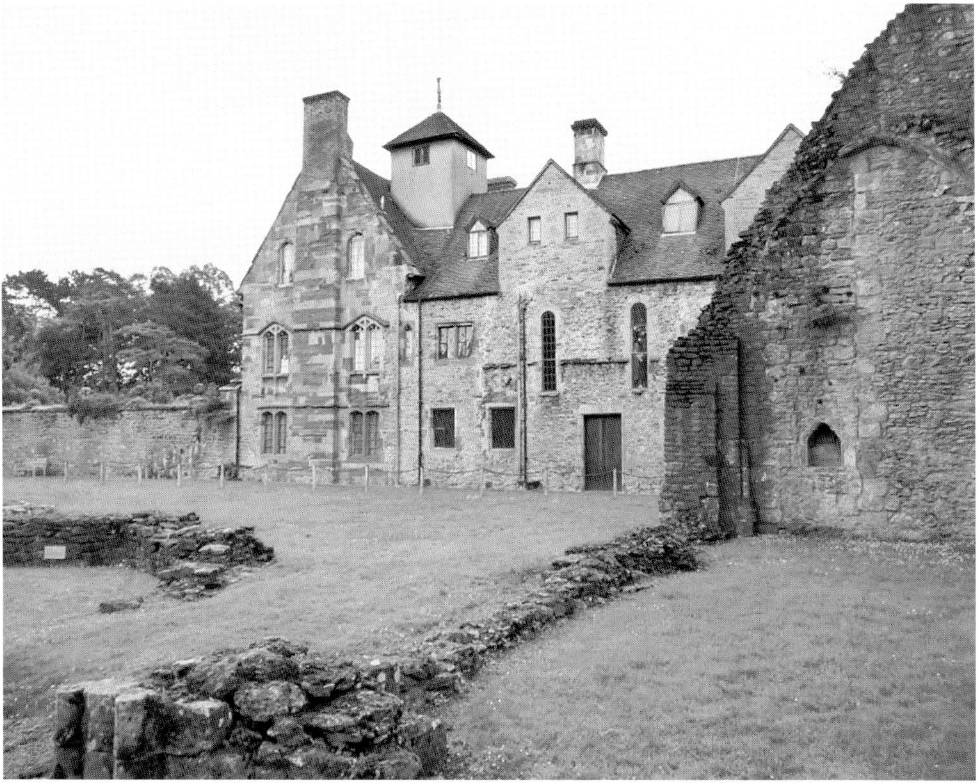

Remains of monastic infirmary at Much Wenlok, Shropshire. The outline of the old infirmary hall can be seen at the forefront of the picture. (Christine Johnstone CC BY-SA 2.0 at geography.co.uk)

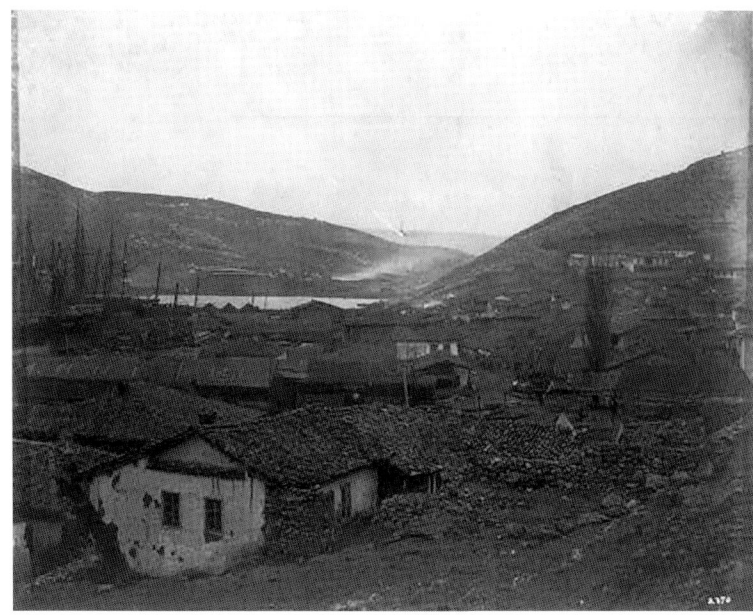

General view of Balaklava Harbour, with the hospital up on the hill, on the right. (Roger Fenton Collection, available at www.loc.gov)

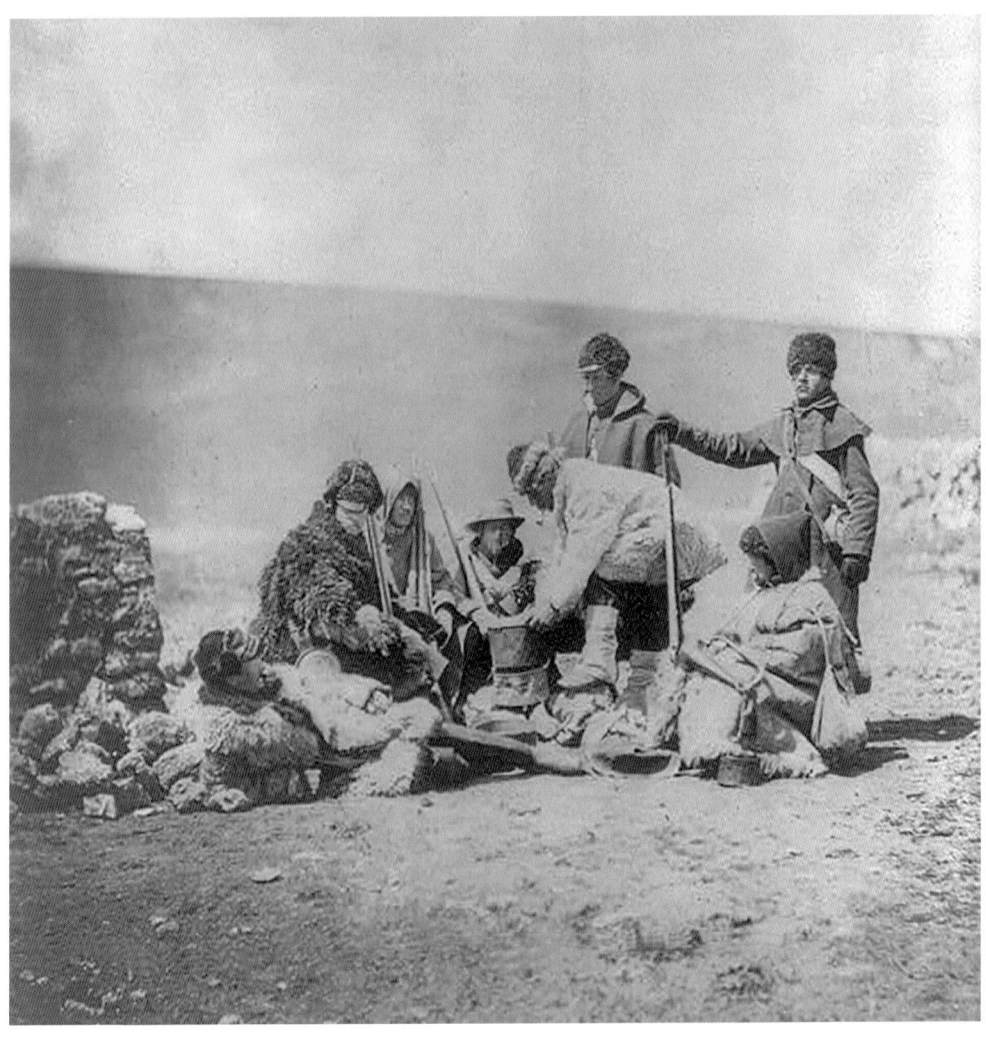

Group of the 47th Regiment in winter dress and ready for the trenches. (Roger Fenton Collection, available at www.loc.gov)

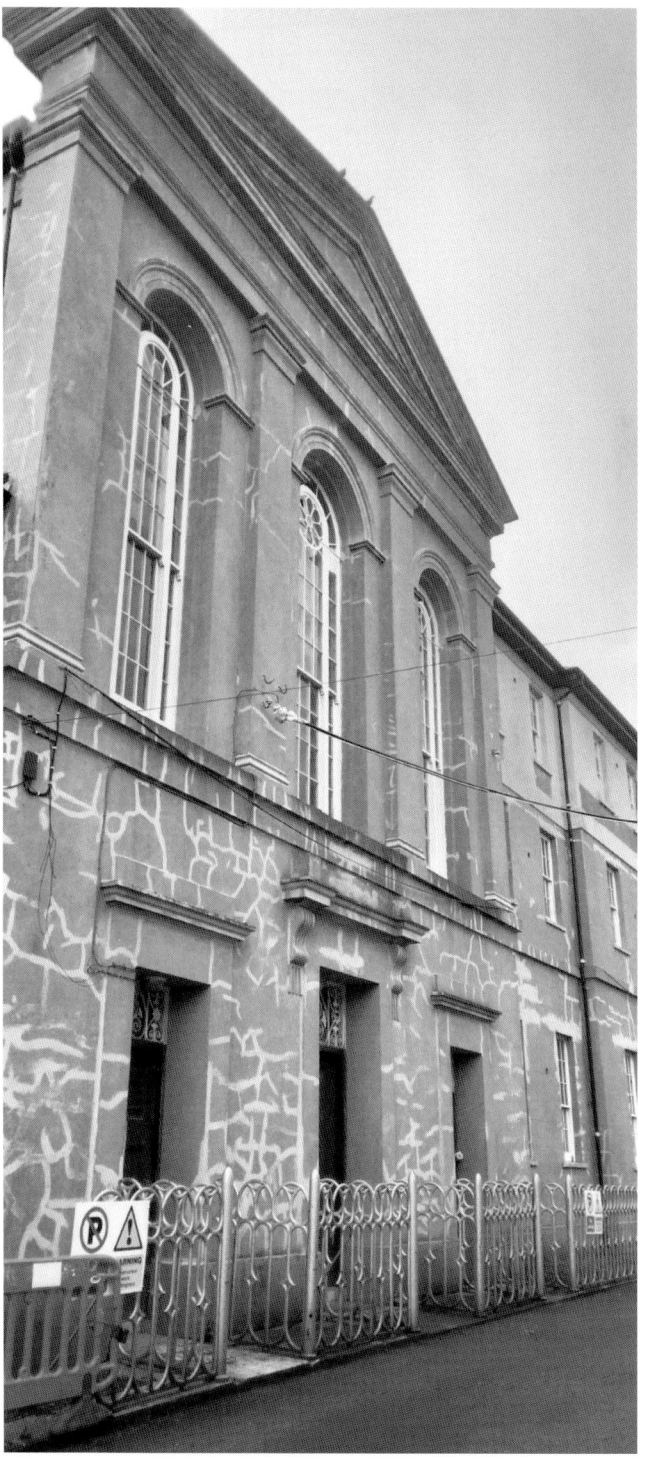

Front of Kinsale Covent in Co. Cork. Now mostly being remodelled and rebuilt for residential properties. (Pauline Caston)

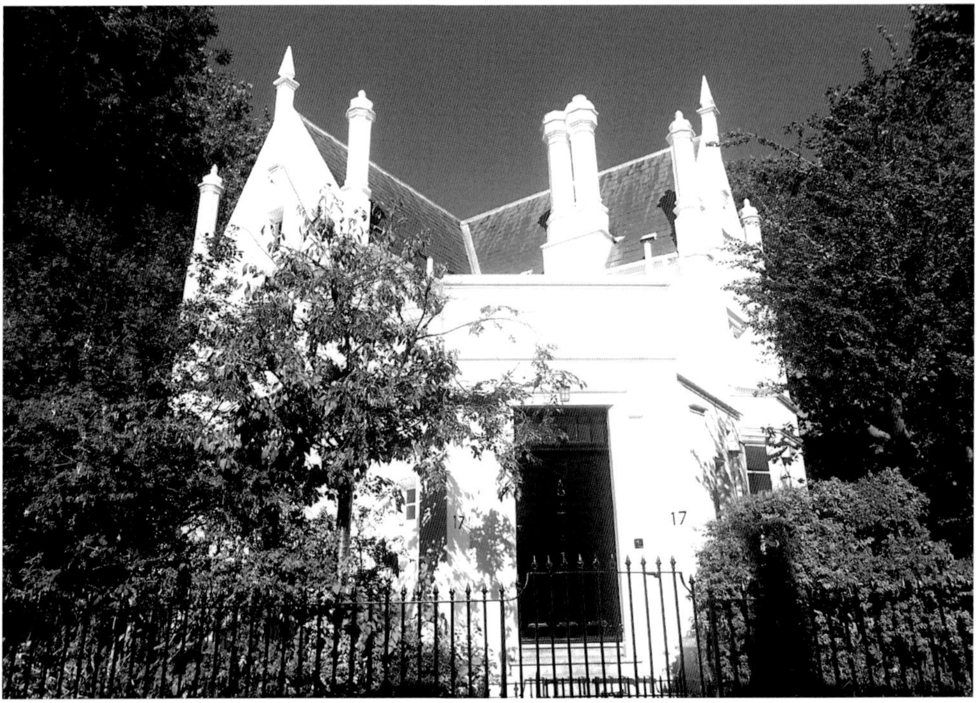

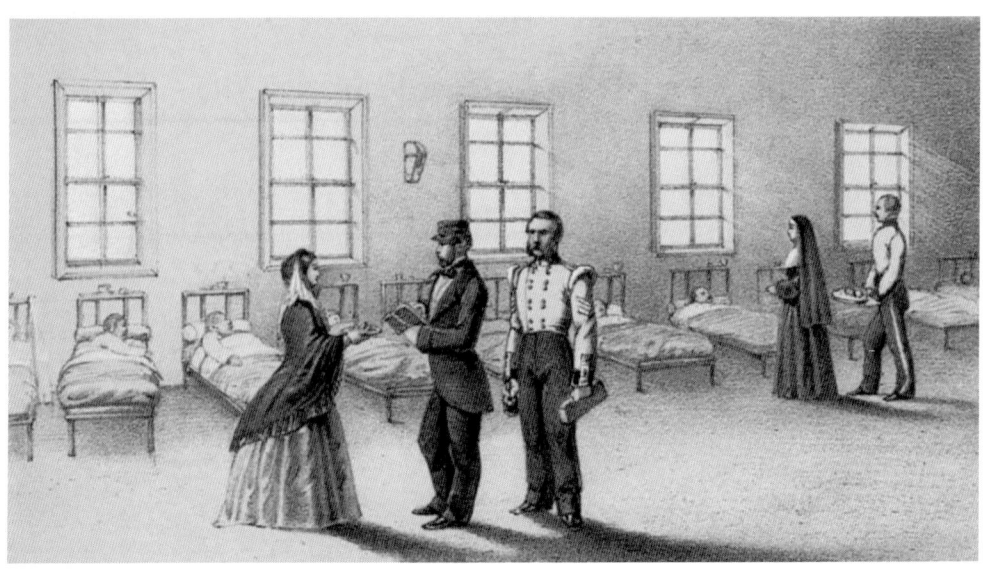

Original dwelling of the first Anglican Sisterhood at 17 Park Village, Regents Park. (Marathon CC BY-SA 2.0 at geograph.co.uk)

Barrack Hospital, Koulali. There is a Sister of Mercy in the background and a Lady Nurse talking to the medical officer. As Florence Nightingale was not at Koulali, this is possibly Mary Stanley as Superintendent and Mother M. Bridgeman. Sketch by a patient. (*Eastern Hospitals and English Nurses: The narrative of twelve months' experience in the hospitals of Koulali and Scutari* by Fanny Taylor)

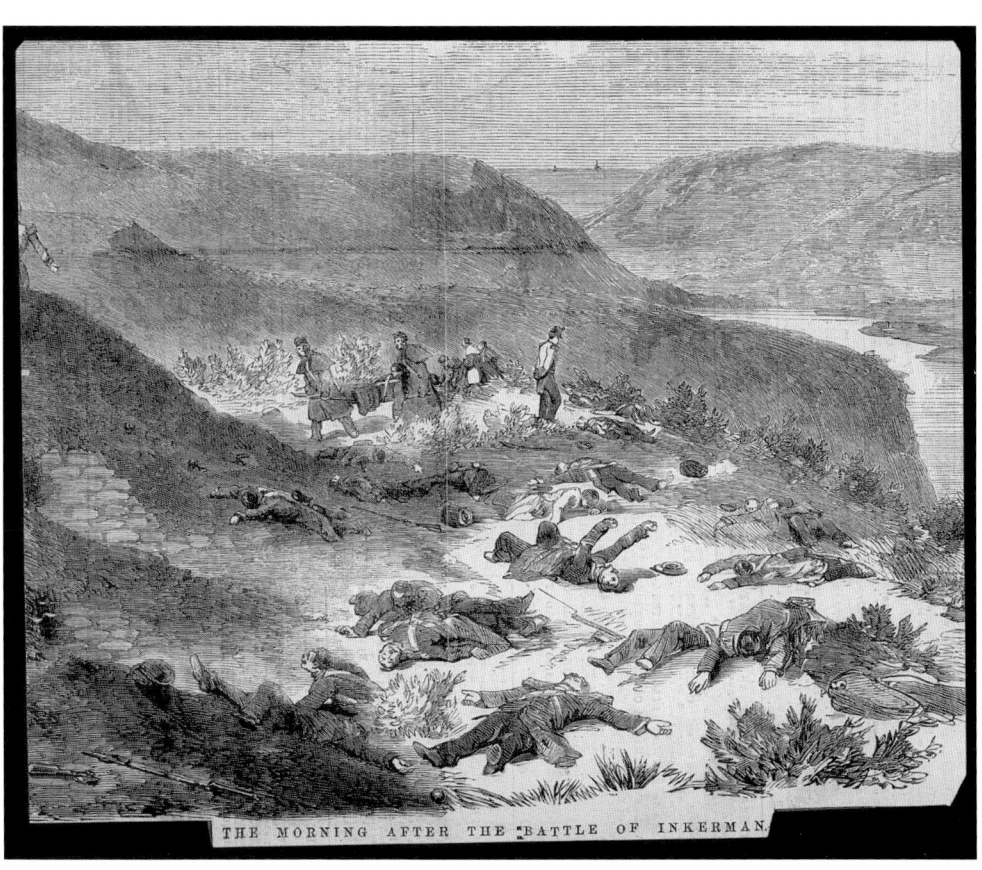

Ambulance men collecting the wounded after the Battle of Inkermann, 1854. (Wellcome Collection)

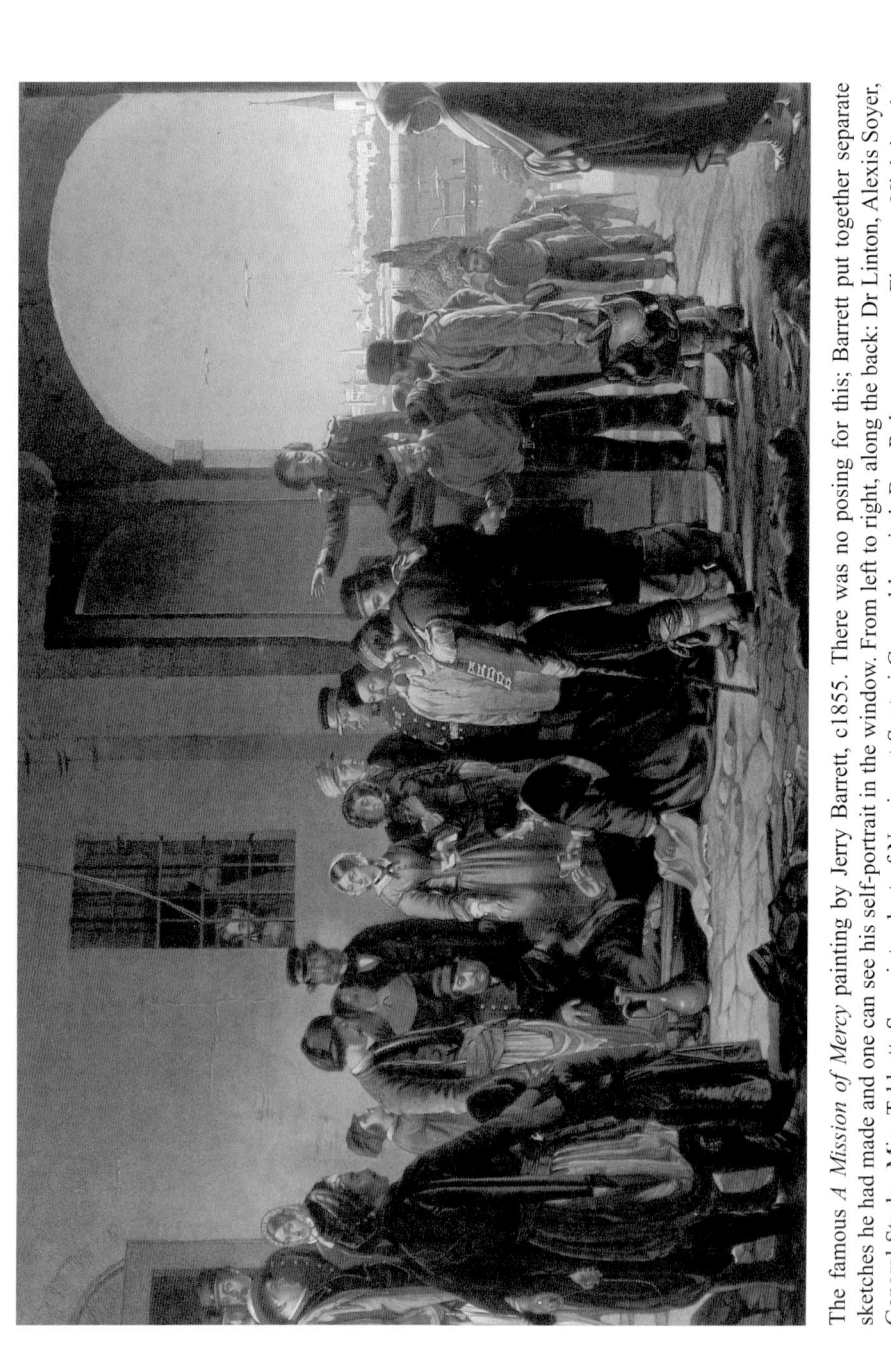

The famous *A Mission of Mercy* painting by Jerry Barrett, c1855. There was no posing for this; Barrett put together separate sketches he had made and one can see his self-portrait in the window. From left to right, along the back: Dr Linton, Alexis Soyer, General Storks, Miss Tebbutt, Superintendent of Nursing at Scutari General hospital, Boy Robert, page to Florence Nightingale, Sister M. Clare Moore, Mother Superior of the English Sisters of Mercy, Dr Cruikshank (kneeling), Colonel Sillery, (the artist is in the window), Florence Nightingale, Mrs Roberts (kneeling), Florence Nightingale's assistant and an experienced nurse, Selena Bracebridge, Charles Bracebridge and Major General Lord William Paulet. (Wellcome Collecton)

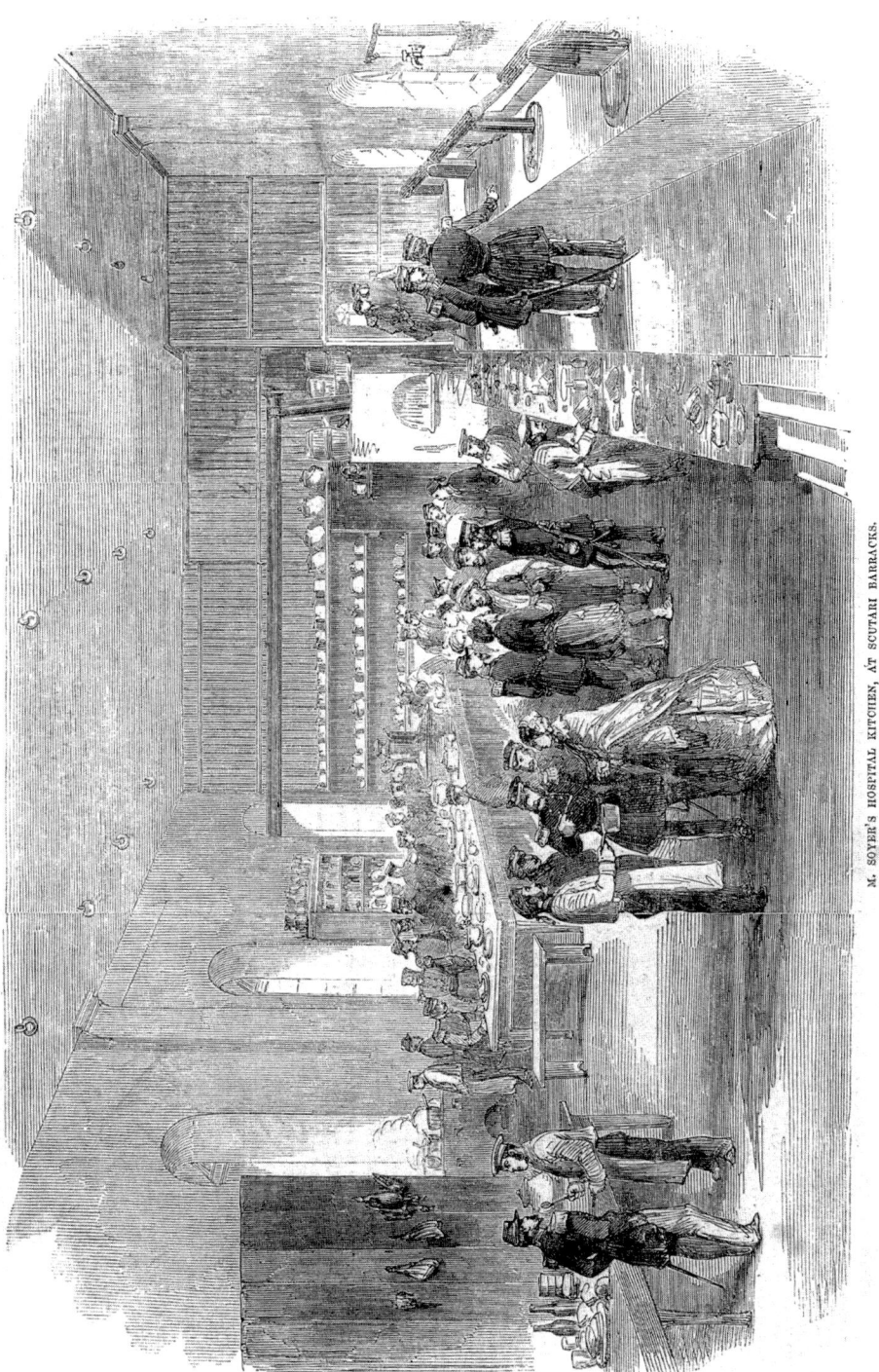

Soyer's kitchen at Scutari Barrack hospital. (Wellcome Collection)

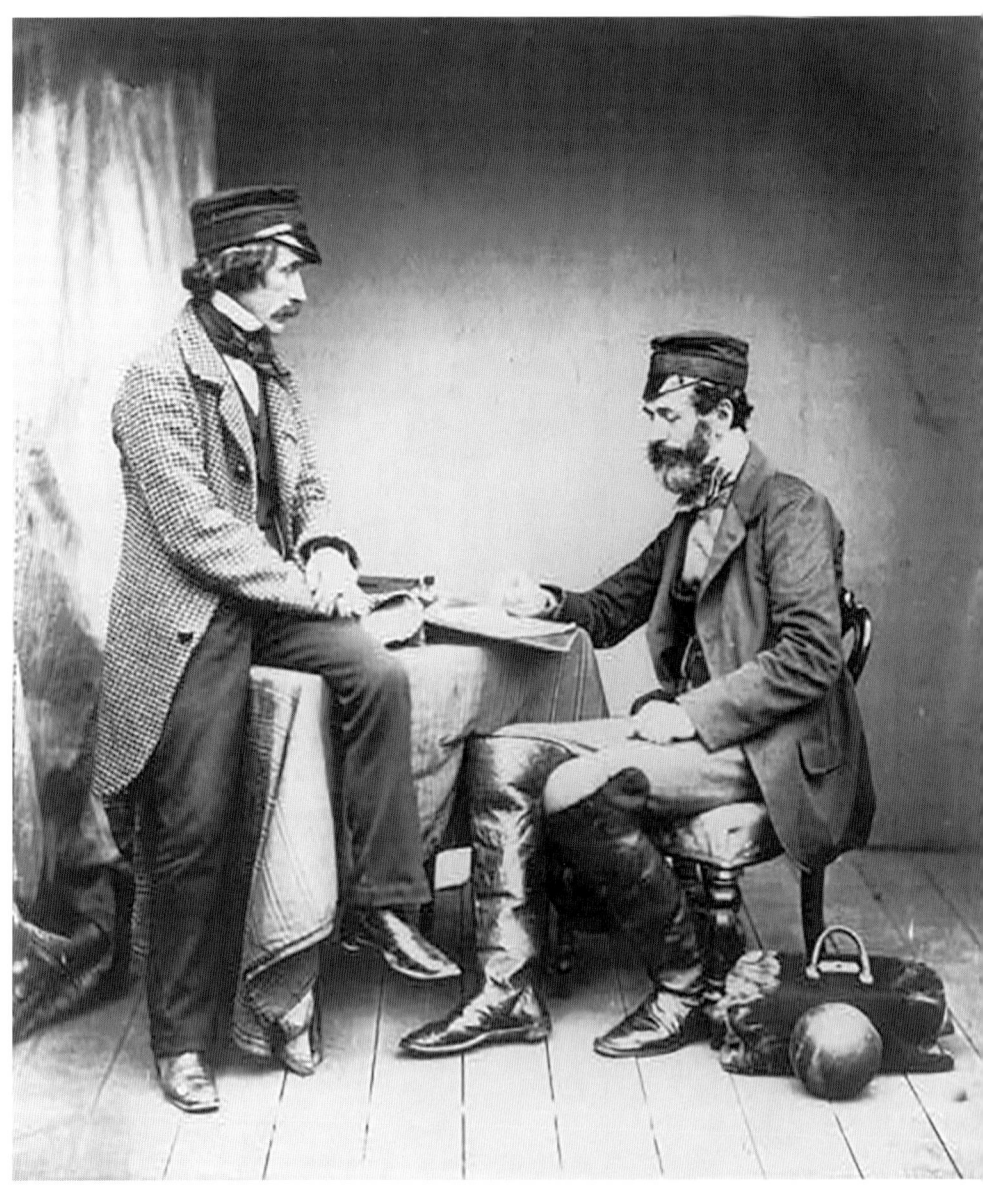

Two members of the Sanitary Commission, March 1855. Sitting on the table, left, is Dr Sutherland, who was to work closely with Florence Nightingale post-Crimea on sanitary reforms. The gentleman sitting down is Sir Robert Rawlinson, engineer and sanitarian. (Roger Fenton Collection, available at www.loc.gov)

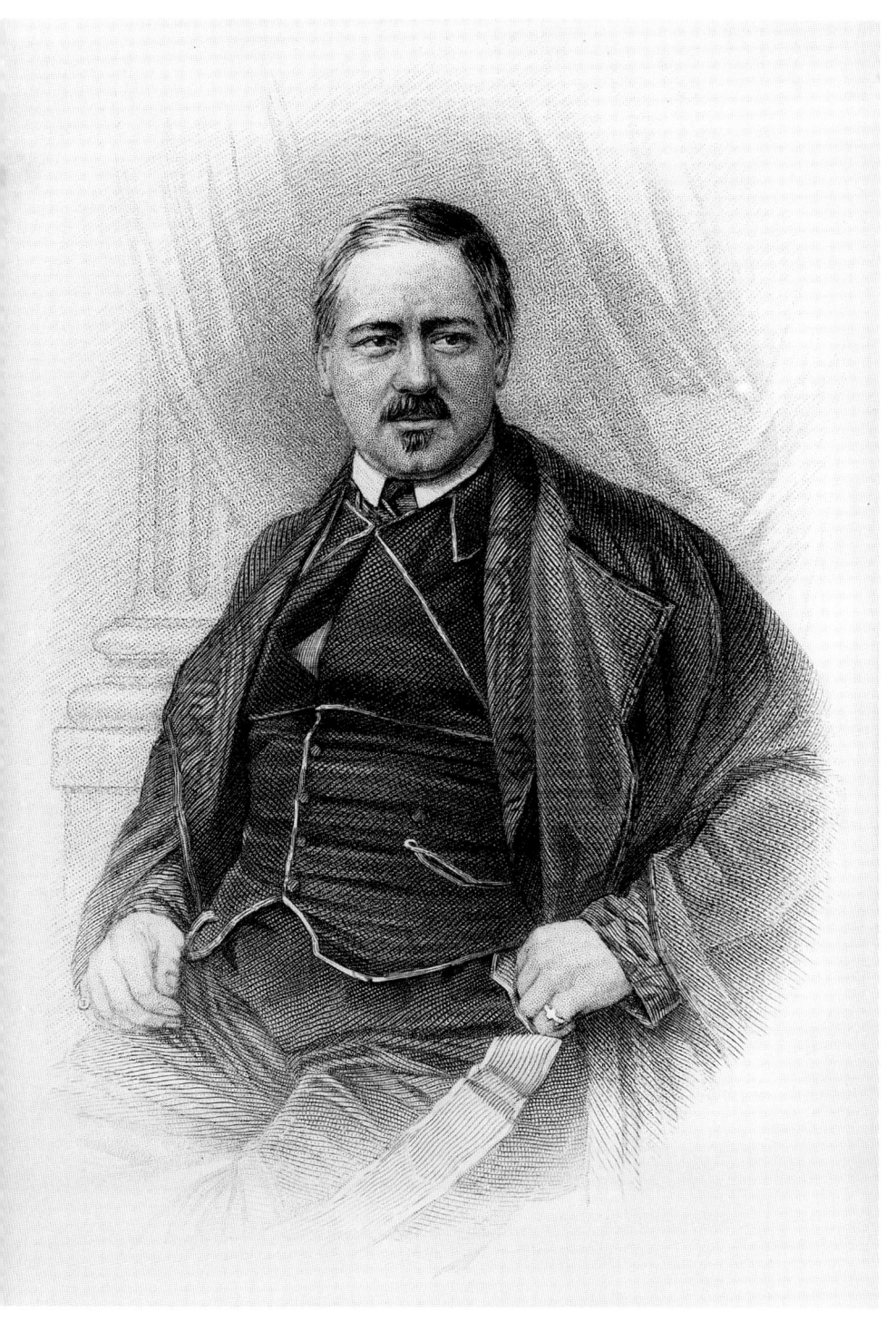

Alexis Soyer, c.1857. (*Soyer's Culinary Campaign*. Wellcome Collection)

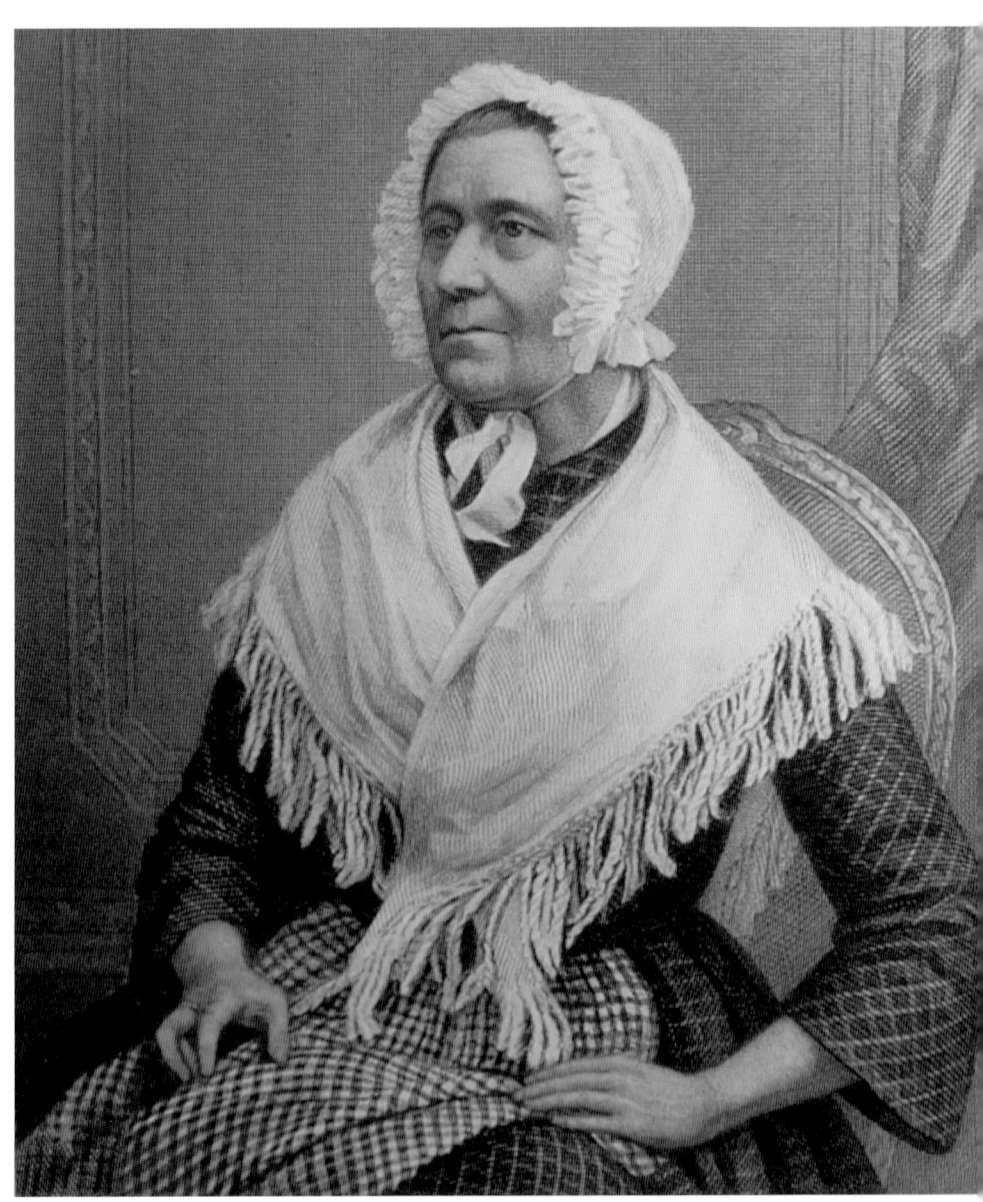
Betsy Cadwaladyr. (British Library)

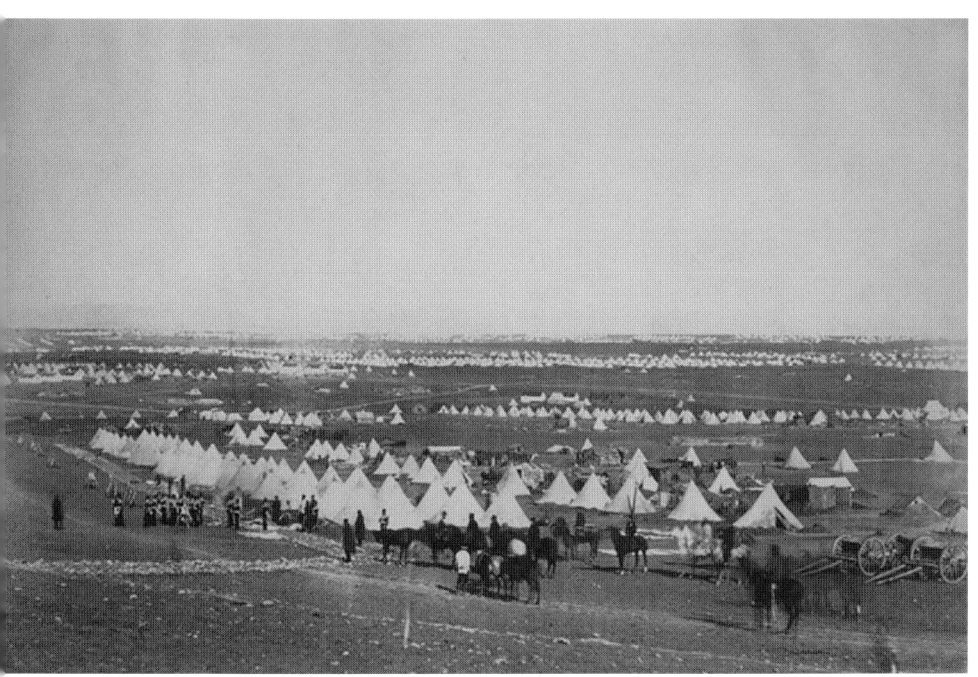

*Above*: Allied camp on the Sebastopol plateau. (Roger Fenton Collection available at www.loc.gov)

*Right*: Dr Sir John Hall. (*The Life and Letters of Sir John Hall.* Archive.org)

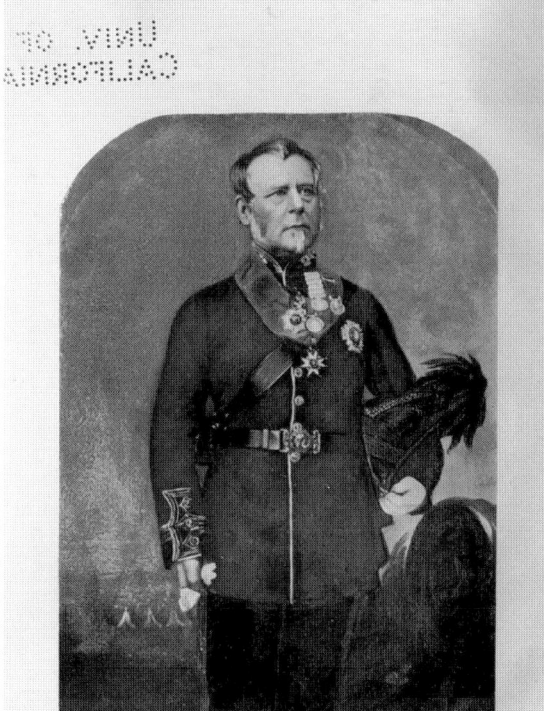

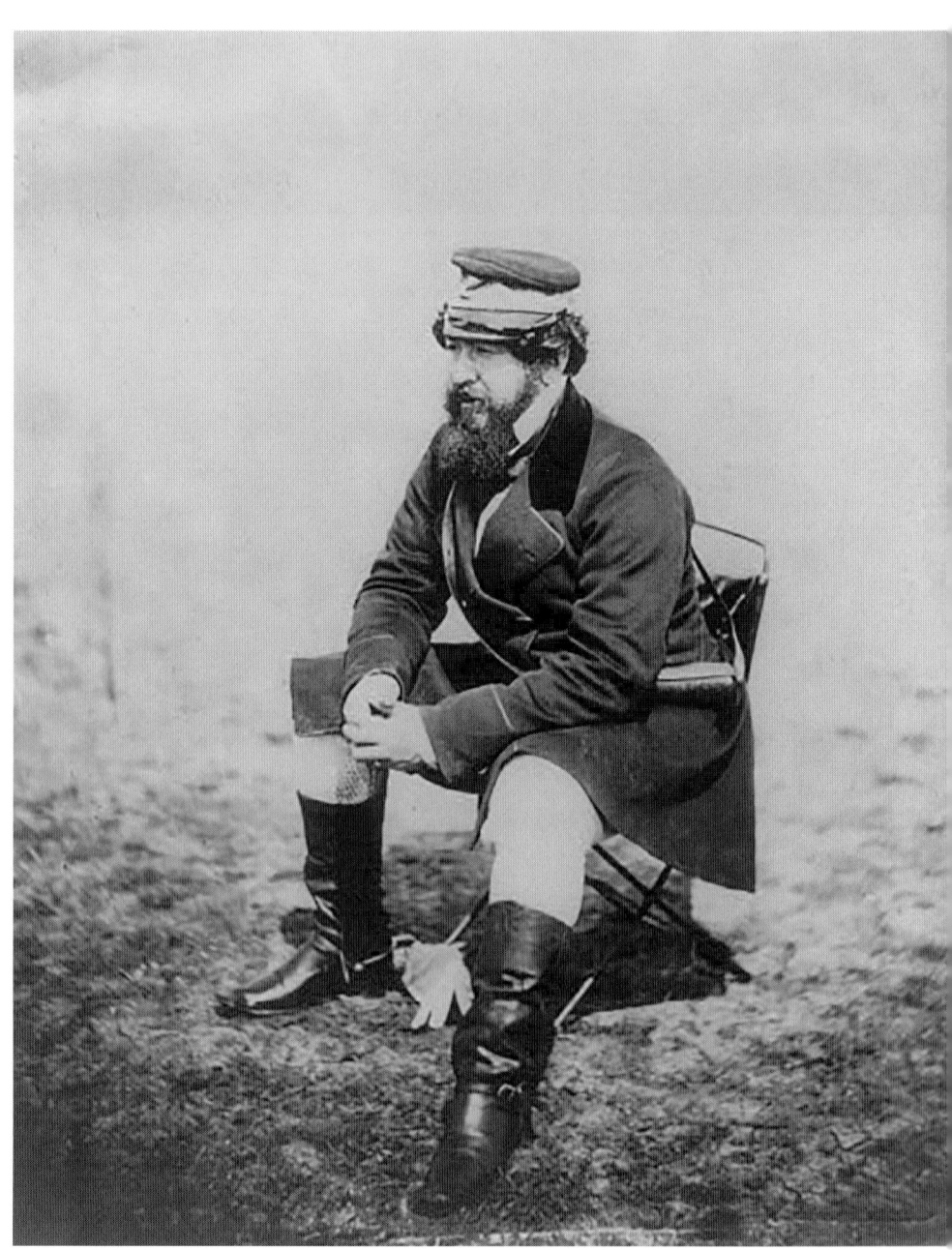

William Russell Howard, the first war correspondent. (Roger Fenton Collection available at www.loc.gov)

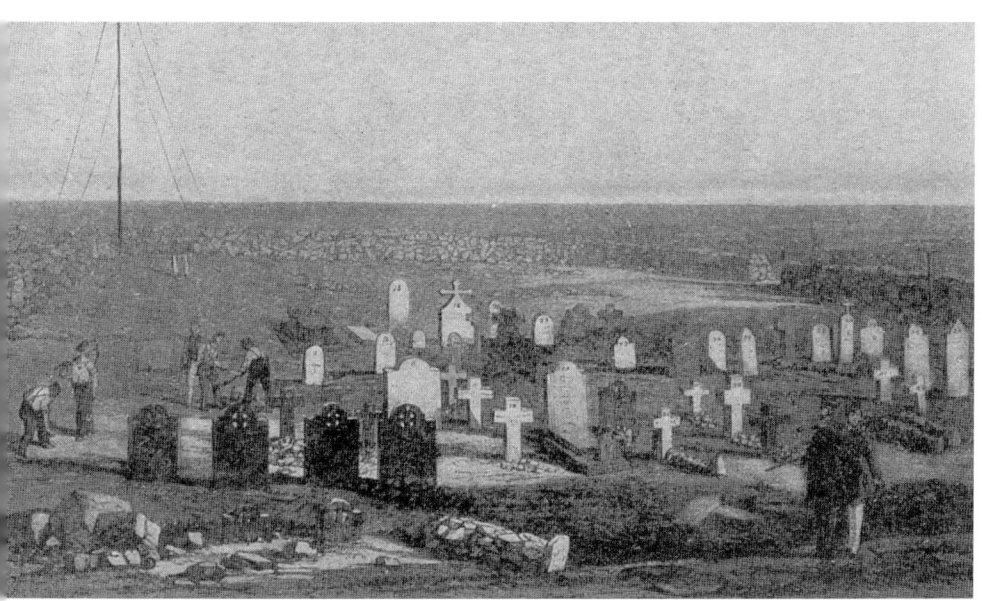

*Above*: Burial ground in the Crimea. (Wellcome Collection)

*Right*: Florence Nightingale. The date on the photograph is 1858, which means it would have been taken between bouts of her post-Crimean illness. (*The Life of Florence Nightingale* by Sir Edward Cook. Archive.org)

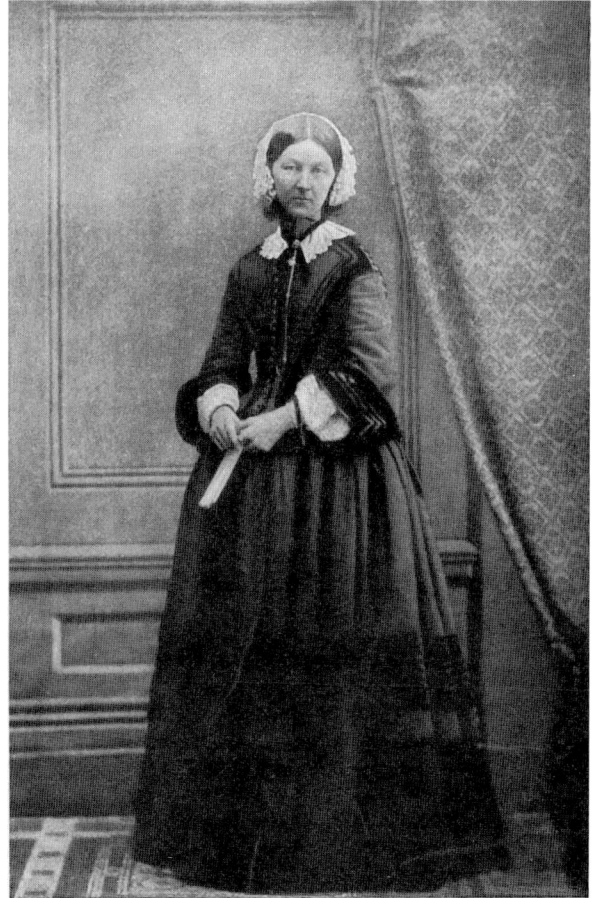

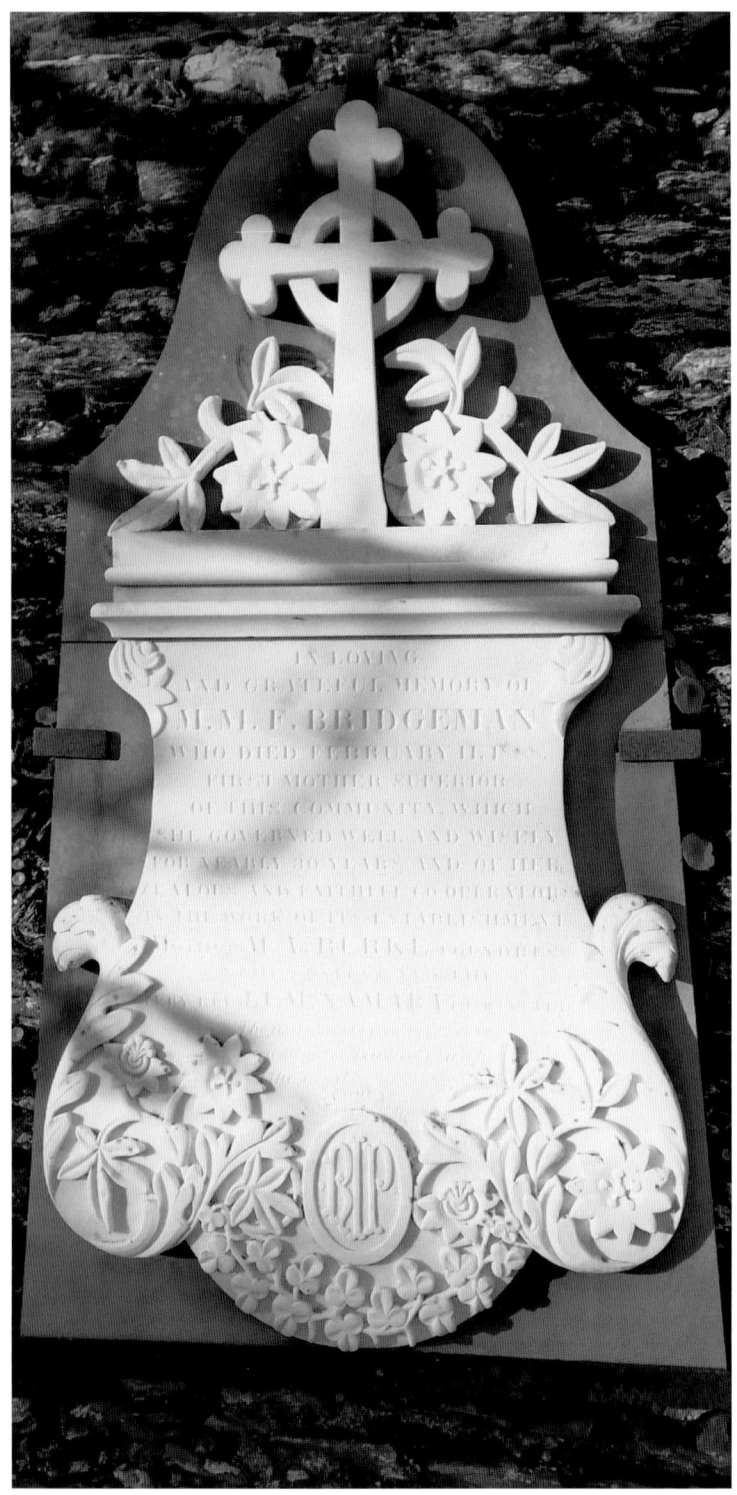

Memorial stone to Mother M. Francis Bridgeman at Kinsale Convent. (Pauline Caston)

# Chapter 6

# RELATIONSHIPS IN THE CRIMEA

*'A French officer, alluding to our Commissariat and other departments, remarked to him that we seemed to follow the system of the middle ages rather than the principles of modern military science, and that his nation regretted our backwardness the more because they saw what noble lives it caused us to sacrifice. This observation was perfectly true, and was made in no hostile spirit.'* Lord Stafford[1]

*'When the war broke out, the French had an organised hospital corps; we had none. We had not even a code of hospital regulations. The whole thing had to be created* denovo *[from new]; and under these disadvantageous circumstances, it is almost wonderful that greater errors have not been committed, and that greater calamities have not occurred.'* Duke of Newcastle[2]

Although this chapter aims to examine the relationships between Mother Bridgeman, Florence Nightingale and Betsy Cadwaladyr, more context needs to be explored around the situation they all found themselves in, the environments they all had to work in and the people they worked with and had to depend upon. Victorian class values (including what we would deem as downright snobbery these days), religious boundaries and mistrust of the Irish Catholics, as well as some myth-busting, also needs to be examined for certain attitudes to be understood and the impact it had on the nursing experiment. For example, Nightingale, as she was unmarried, still needed her parents' permission to leave for the Crimea, despite being 34 years old and an experienced nurse by this time![3]

## The Irish, Catholicism and Religious Connotations

In September 1850, Pope Pius IX issued *Universalis Ecclesiae,* a papal bull announcing the revival of a Catholic diocese hierarchy, something that had vanished shortly after Elizabeth I took the throne in 1558. The bull was met with horror and hostility and labelled the 'Papal Aggression'. This attitude can be attributed to a couple of schools of thought, first of which was a large increase of Irish immigrants to England in the first half of the nineteenth century. On the back of the great tragedy that was the Irish Famine came an influx of destitute Irish. Before the Crimean War began at the end of 1853, the Irish-born population of England, Scotland and Wales rose from 415,000 in 1841 to 727,000 in 1851 and the Irish would account for 3.5 per cent of the population by 1861. The Irish were already considered an inferior race at this point by both upper and lower classes and the socio-economic hardship of the 1840s in England meant there was much hatred aimed at them – and therefore Catholicism – by the time of the start of the Crimean War. Secondly, politically-driven dialogue between the years 1835 – 1850 accused Catholicism of being dangerous (the religion of age-old enemies of England such as France and Spain) and faithful only to a foreign power (Rome). Ergo, Catholics could not be loyal citizens and were dominated by the priesthood, whether you were Irish or not.[4] The Bermondsey Convent of the Sisters of Mercy was the first Irish convent domiciled in England in 1839, the first to do so since Henry VIII's Reformation in the mid-sixteenth century. Five Sisters of Mercy from Bermondsey left England for the Crimea in the early hours of 17 October 1854 ahead of any other nursing volunteers after a plea to the Sisterhood from the Bishop of Southwark, Dr Grant, on 14 October.[5] Although requested to await FN's arrival in Paris, there was to be much suspicion around these Irish Sisters and the Catholic chaplains during the campaign.

Before any nurses went to the Crimea, the leading Irish newspaper of the day, *The Freeman's Journal,* published an editorial piece in August 1854 about the dearth of Roman Catholic chaplains in the British Army. At that point, the article states that out of the approximate 30,000 troops, one-third were Irish Catholics and had but two priests for their spiritual needs, including the dying man, be it from gunshot or disease. The article goes onto say that Popery was not expected in a military camp, but that Roman Catholic soldiers who were accepted for service in the British military should be allowed to have their spiritual instruction.[6] This was not a new thing; five months earlier, in March 1854, Sidney Herbert had explained this during a House of Commons sitting:

> It was perfectly true ... that the Roman Catholic soldiers amounted in round numbers to about one-third of the whole Army ... he was not aware of the numbers as they existed at particular stations. This, however, had nothing to do with the matter, because, in the relief which annually took place, and the shifting of regiments from one station to another, the relative proportions of Protestants and Roman Catholics at each place must, of course, be constantly shifting also. At one time there might be a Highland regiment, composed in greater part of Presbyterians, and in the next year the same station might be occupied by another with a large proportion of Roman Catholics; and therefore any argument founded upon the particular numbers occupying a particular station at any given moment would be entirely fallacious, because the numbers themselves were fluctuating and temporary.[7]

Demands for an increase in Catholic chaplains had been waging for at least fifty years before the Crimean War; the Army Chaplains

Department was founded in 1796 and was purely Anglican. Dr Grant, Bishop of Southwark and son of a Waterloo veteran who had spent much of his childhood following the regiments, had been campaigning with the government since 1852 for more religious and spiritual instruction for both soldiers in the army and sailors in the navy. Grant was aware of treading a fine line and not to rock the political boat regarding Catholicism, but Sidney Herbert had informed Grant in February 1854 that arrangements had been made for two Catholic chaplains to leave with the 10,000 Catholic soldiers who made up the 26,000 Crimean Expeditionary Force.[8]

Although the Catholic Church requested a priest should accompany Bridgeman's Sisters of Mercy on their departure, the War Office disagreed, especially as the Bermondsey Sisters, who had travelled out with FN a month earlier, did not have one. A regulation code was thus drawn up in Dublin, the first two items stating that 'The Sisters shall attend to the spiritual and material needs of the Catholic soldiers in the hospitals; but to the material needs only of non-Catholics' and 'They shall not discuss religious topics with those outside the Catholic church. If a desire for knowledge of Catholic doctrine is evinced, they shall inform the chaplain.' Mother Bridgeman was also made the head of their spiritual guidance at this time.[9]

The question of proselytism was raised in the House of Commons just days after the arrival of the Sisters of Mercy; Sidney Herbert was questioned on the use of Scripture Readers being sent to the Crimea, where they were refused entry into the hospitals. He asked why were the Sisters of Mercy and other religious orders '… whose duty and object it was to promulgate their own religious opinions, were admitted into the hospitals. Considering that the majority of our soldiers were Protestants, he wished to know whether this report was well founded …' Scripture Readers had been working the with Army since 1838, sending out ex-military personnel and men of good standing within Christianity to work with chaplains supporting the soldiers. Sidney Herbert explained, under questioning, that just as troops were made up from all denominations, including Catholics,

Church of England, Protestants etc., and that all must be considered good Christians, then so were the women who had all volunteered to nurse for the health of the army and had agreed to rules as such. Herbert acknowledged Scripture Readers had been sent out but that a few of them had decided to enter the hospitals without permission and spread controversial religious ideals '... that was evidently in violation of the rules of the hospital, and the proceedings which had consequently been taken, he felt bound to say, were absolutely necessary for the purpose of carrying out the regulations of the hospital ...'[10]

This was just the beginning of such accusations for the Sisters of Mercy. In the early months of 1855, Sister Doyle, in her diary, notes that most of the Protestant clergy were friendly, polite and that many became friends with the Sisters. However, Doyle also noted how they received letters from the War Office complaining of the Sisters interfering with the Protestant soldiers and knew that certain chaplains were watching their every move. Doyle, however, says that they '... found the Protestant soldiers respectful and grateful as we could desire.'[11]

Certain chaplains were indeed watching their every move, especially the senior Anglican chaplain to the forces, Mr J.E. Sabin, who had been in post before the arrival of FN and her nurses. In February 1855, a Sister of Mercy was accused of converting a Protestant soldier to Catholicism at Koulali Hospital. This was investigated by Mary Stanley and it was found that the young soldier had requested to speak to a Catholic priest (Father Ronan), who then asked a Sister (Sister M. Elizabeth) to instruct the young man, who had felt he was in the wrong religion as his family were mainly Catholics. This episode of assumed proselytising was mentioned in FN's biography by Cook[12] and in a letter dated 15 February 1855 from FN to Herbert.[13] Cook, unfortunately, fails to mention that there was no basis for these accusations and Sabin ended up back-tracking slightly.[14] By June 1855, Sabin was demanding a monthly report from Father Ronan to detail where Ronan conducted his administration, the number of Catholics under Ronan's care per month, the number of services held by Ronan and any remarks he deemed interesting and/or important. This was quickly rebuffed by Father Michael Cuffe, senior Catholic Chaplain: 'I am not aware of any military law which orders me, or any of my brother Roman Catholic Chaplains, to give in any reports or returns to the Protestant Chaplain-General; and until I am made aware of such a law, I must decline complying with the request made in your letter ...'[15] Sabin was eventually censured by Lord Panmure for religious intolerance and invalided home shortly after this letter in June 1855; in a letter to the Bracebridges in August 1855, FN states that 'Mr Sabin is ill and gone home. He is no loss to me ...'[16]

By September 1855, there seems to be disgruntlement that the Sisters of Mercy are consistently attending to the spiritual needs of the Catholic soldiers, despite this adhering exactly to the agreement made with the War Office when they had departed ten months previously – that is what they were allowed to do. FN's letter to Lady Canning dated 9 September 1855 complained that the Roman Catholics now instruct *all* of their own faith and the '2nd party of Nuns who came out now wander over the whole Hospital out of Nursing hours, not confining themselves to their own wards nor even to Patients, but ... groups of Orderlies & Convalescents in the Corridors – doing the work of ten Chaplains ... while they quote the words of the W[ar] Office which indeed seem to have been left intentionally vague ...'[17] Damned if you do, damned if you don't! Overall, twenty-three Catholic Chaplains served during the Crimean War, five of whom died in service. Within a year of the end of the war in 1856, the government expanded the numbers of the Army Chaplain's Department, across all Anglican, Catholic and Presbyterian denominations.[18]

## A Matter of Class

A very loose framework but one with a clear definition of Victorian class structure combines the upper, middle and lower/working classes. Upper classes, headed by the monarch, included dukes, duchesses, earls, ladies and lords. Wealth was never in doubt and a top education expected. Middle classes, those of earned wealth, grew steadily and included professions such as doctors and engineers and some evolved into the middle-upper classes early on. The Industrial Revolution progressed their standing in society and around the year 1842, accounted for one-sixth of the population. Working classes had a sub-division of the 'under-class'; the gap between skilled and unskilled labourer. Both middle and upper classes were influenced by variables such as power and how much they imposed their will on others; prestige and associations with social standings, lifestyles and individual qualities; wealth, including properties, land, livestock. Only the working class had no influence on politics and continued in a cycle of poverty, lack of education and, at the very worst, ended up in the workhouse.[19]

The Victorian values of the class system would impact the nursing in the Crimea. For an example, as early as 1830, Sir James Paget, the famous surgeon, pathologist and discoverer of Paget's Disease, at St Bart's in London stated that nurses were 'dull, unobservant and untaught women', whilst another hospital preferred to recruit 'old women of the charwoman class' to nurse.[20] This may go some way to explain the initial hostility between the working class Betsy and the middle-upper-class FN. Crimean doctors did not escape class prejudice either; Lord Palmerston, who became prime minister in 1855, and whose country estate in Hampshire bordered that of the Nightingales, thus socially connecting both families, stated post-Crimean War that the failings of the Medical Department (as well as the Commissariat and Transport Service) would not have existed had the departments been run by the gentry and/or the aristocracy.[21] However, a speech in parliament in December 1854 by Colonel Dunne stated that

> ... He [Colonel Dunne] admitted that the Commissariat had latterly done its duty well, but it was badly served at first.

On this head he would not bear hardly on the Government; for he would admit that the long peace had made it extremely difficult to get together an organised corps of officers perfectly competent by training and experience for such peculiar duties as the Commissariat had to perform, and great allowance for their shortcomings ought, therefore, to be made. With regard to the medical department; it was a mistake not to attach the medical officers to the brigades in the first instance, as their services would thus have been rendered much more speedily and effectively available. Officers and stores were sent out in abundance by the Government; unfortunately, the stores did not reach their destination, and there was so much confusion that the stores were in one place and the wounded in another. Again, when the army landed at the Crimea, the Government had not prepared proper reserves.[22]

It is worth noting that Palmerston was also an absentee landlord of vast estates in Western Ireland and had evicted 2,000 of his tenants during the Great Famine, although he had financed some of his tenants on their one-way journey to Canada. By 1854, the Duke of Newcastle was the Secretary *for* War (a new position created for the Crimean War) whilst Sidney Herbert was Secretary *at* War. Herbert acted as a type of assistant but stepped up in the emergency created by the Crimea War, assisting the overworked duke and utilising his keen interest in the care of the sick. Both were acquainted with Nightingale in social circles in which they all partook.[23]

At the time of the Crimean War, because the army medical services were so antiquated, social status topped skill in that officers tended to be aristocrats and/or wealthy individuals who could simply buy their commission. A debate on the condition and conduct of the Army on 29 January 1855 in the House of Commons saw the MP for Middlesex, Secretary for the Admiralty and former military Officer, Mr Bernal Osborne, question the morality of only the wealthy being able to buy their commissions for the army, no matter the lack of talent, and that anyone who had the skill set and talents needed for an undertaking such as the Crimea, were simply discredited because they could not afford it. He questioned that

> If we are to have any reform in the British army, with a stern hand you must do away with the practice, and put the whole staff arrangements on a different footing ... I have been told it is not proper for a person in my situation to speak; but, in my mind, the safety of our whole army is at stake. If you constitute another army on the same footing, I do not think it will do any better. It is not enough that they should win battles, they must go through campaigns; and we have seen the lamentable and disgraceful way in which this war has been conducted. I say, in this, I impute no inefficiency to the men. They are the victims of the system, and this House is to blame for having so long submitted to it. We were warned of this long ago.

The wealthy individuals in charge, in turn looked down upon the regimental surgeons who had to depend upon the regimental colonel for their supplies, resources and had no authoritative control even over their own patients and the orderlies. Even the Director General had no authority over the regimental surgeons; this was Dr Andrew Smith and, along with Dr John Hall (both highly qualified doctors), became scapegoats of the press, the public and FN regarding the utter disaster of that first winter in the Crimea.

Andrew Smith (1797 – 1872), had worked his way up from a working-class background; interestingly, he was also a Catholic, so straight away you have two traits looked down upon in upper Victorian society. He was the son of a Border farm shepherd in Roxburghshire who, after attending a local school, became a surgeon's apprentice and studied medicine at the University of Edinburgh. In August 1815 he joined the Army Medical Service and was granted M.D in 1819. In 1820 he was sent to South Africa as a medical assistant attached to the 72nd Regiment and ended up staying there for sixteen years, becoming a scientist, renowned zoologist and naturist as well as continuing to supervise medical personnel. He of all people would understand the need of medical care in the field of war zones and his initial attempts in preparing for the Crimean War show this. When he returned to England in 1836, he became a staff surgeon within the army and five years later, in 1841, was promoted to Principal Medical Officer at the medical services HQ in Fort Pitt, Chatham, Kent. He married in 1844 and in 1845 became Professional Assistant to Sir James McGrigor, Director General of the Medical Department, and within a year became his deputy. McGrigor retired in February 1851 with Smith promoted to his position and two years later, in February 1853, Smith became Director General of Army and Ordnance Medical Departments.[24]

Dr Andrew Smith, although described as a 'man of forceful character and irascible and pugnacious temper' by his Royal College of Physicians biography, was also described as being reserved, abrupt but of 'great integrity ... indefatigable'.[25] His career is one of success and he is somebody who could have easily been replaced by either the Secretary for War, the Duke of Newcastle, or Sidney Herbert. But this was not the case. FN made up her mind that he was the enemy due to the conditions she found upon arrival at Scutari, but he had relied on reports from his principal medical officers as he was to remain in London throughout the war. In a letter to Sidney Herbert on 4 January 1855, FN described him as '... that old smoke-dried Dr Andrew Smith who is the God of the Officials here ...'[26] However, this was partly due to her frustrations at not being able to purvey the simplest things; she had tried at the end of December 1854 to obtain flannel shirts, socks and drawers for the soldiers, items deemed urgently important by Smith's own Deputy Inspector-General Dr David Dumbreck when surveying the area in April 1854. FN also requested plates, tin cups, earthenware urine pots, bedpans, stools and tea pails. Unfortunately, all that was available to her on 31 December 1854 were some teapots, coffee pots, metal urine pots, a few bedpans, some stools with broken frames but no clothing.[27]

Dr Andrew Smith was not notified to mobilise the medical department until 10 February 1854 and afterwards wasted no time; on 18 February he wrote on the necessity of field ambulances. On 3 March 1854 he had designed waggons to act as ambulances and this was put in motion. However, Smith also recommended (but was not responsible for) men from Chatham: '400 men, at the least, of good character, to be always present with the waggons'. Although he was denied permission to take 400 men from Chatham himself, he was told that Colonel Tulloch and Colonel Maule (the same Lauderdale Maule of whom Martha Clough declared her love for, and who denied FN's authority and went to nurse in the Highland Regiment's hospital, with hope of visiting his grave) had arranged that the ambulance corps would be manned by military pensioners of whom the Secretary at War, the Duke of Newcastle, had overall responsibility. Smith vehemently opposed this, claiming his five years at Chatham saw him invalid 20,000 men and he knew from experience that these pensioners would not be capable of the duties required of them.

On 4 April, Smith wrote to the office of Lord Raglan, Commander in Chief of the British Army at the time. He wrote about his concerns regarding the state of the roads and difficulties in conveyance of injured troops off the fields. Smith suggested

> This assistance may be variously supplied; but feeling as I do, that it will never be willingly conceded in the shape of able-bodied soldiers, I at once, in order to get rid of all difficulties, propose that a hospital corps for the object be raised immediately the army reaches Turkey, and that is all consist of at least 800 natives (Armenians), if possible and shall be under regular military discipline.

Smith recommended sending Dr Frederick Brett, who could speak several local languages and had resided in Constantinople for several years. His letter was initially ignored, although the War Office eventually sent out Dr Brett, who found no military support and was sent home by Raglan. On 11 May 1854, Smith again submitted guidance on hospital ships, including ships to bring those back to England who could no longer fight, ships stationed in the harbour and those to care for the sick if hospitals ended up being established away from army stations (which they were). He gave instructions that berths should be high-decked, allowing for proper ventilation and having fixed beds; when capacity had been reached, the ship would sail either home or its fate decided on by local authority. This letter was never replied to and 'Dr Smith supposed that, having tendered advice, he had no further authority to insist upon what he thought absolutely necessary'.[28]

## Interdisciplinary relationships that did not work

What did happen in July 1854 was that the War Office sent out 370 retired military pensioners, of whom 260 were to work as orderlies/stretcher-bearers, and 110 as waggon drivers. It was a disastrous action, mainly due to alcohol, disease and death; not long after arrival, many found the work duties too heavy, as well as succumbing to illness and the dreaded cholera. Very soon, with little control or guidance from their captain, only sixty of the 270 were able to perform any duties, although that was when they were not incapacitated from drink. It only took a few weeks for the so-called Ambulance Corps to be on the very edge of non-existence, and this was the nearest thing to nurse staffing before FN and subsequent female nurses arrived.[29]

The need for an efficient system of orderlies was nothing new. In 1819, John Millingen (1782 – 1862), an army surgeon who had been the principal surgeon of cavalry at the Battle of Waterloo, wrote an Army Officer's Manual regarding medical care whilst in the theatre of war, advising the need for an ambulance corps: 'The personal talents and efforts of medical officers will however prove of little or no avail, if they have not proper and sufficient assistance in the field; not afforded on the spur of the moment, and in the hurry and tumult of war, but formed and organised upon a systematic and liberal plan.' His plan formation included details of attachments such as farriers and wheelwrights, waggon design and supplies. His recommendations were put aside, however, and the failure to form something from these suggestions came back to haunt those in charge in 1854.[30]

It was Dr Andrew Smith who, by December 1854, had consulted with the Secretary for War, Henry Pelham-Clinton, 5th Duke of Newcastle, along with George Guthrie, an eminent London surgeon and veteran of the Peninsular War and Waterloo who had significantly reduced battlefield injuries. Guthrie had also helped implement a highly efficient Army Medical Service forty years previous to the Crimea.[31] After consulting both these knowledgeable men, the Duke of Newcastle consequently increased numbers and in December 1854 gave a speech in parliament:

> I consulted with Dr. Smith—the head of the medical department—who was adverse to an increase of the regimental surgeons, and who was of opinion that the best mode of strengthening the medical department was by adding to the medical staff, and not to the regimental surgeons; experience having shown, as he stated, that the greatest requirements were in the hospitals, where the regimental surgeons were not available ... The staff was, therefore, increased, as was recommended by Dr. Smith, and the regimental staff was increased in the mode pointed out by Mr. Guthrie.[32]

Although a unified Army Medical Corps was formed in June 1855, it did not arrive in the Crimea until the November, and although this action has been attributed to the letters of FN to Sidney Herbert, most notably a couple of letters from January 1855, we have seen how it was not a new request. In her letters to Herbert, FN details hospital systems she developed from her pre-Crimean working knowledge of medical professionals and nursing needs, as well as her hands-on Crimean experience; most importantly, she could detail the rationale of her suggestions. FN requested ward masters, a steward, and an efficient system of orderlies, not the system currently in place where the orderlies were usually convalescing soldiers who were then sent back to their regiments, or soldiers whose regiment deemed them next to useless, and who all liked too much alcohol.[33] One of the nursing Anglican Sisters described orderlies in the Scutari hospital as unfeeling, impatient, inconsistent and of inferior character. The Sisters of Mercy noted this too, with Bridgeman stating that, 'The orderlies lost their perquisites and they were all the more sober for it ...' After witnessing so many distressing deaths by cholera, Sister Mary Aloysius said, 'The orderlies are indifferent as to life or death'. Betsy describes the Ambulance Corps as '... tipsy fellows, and ate and drank the supplies which they ought to have carried to the patients'.[34]

FN compared this deficient system to that of the French, who had an efficient Orderly Corps and, as we have seen, this was not a new problem. It had been an issue from a medical point of view and largely overlooked until December 1854; at this point, Sidney Herbert had been liaising with Dr Andrew Smith already, admitting the complete failure of the hospital orderlies who were '... rude, uneducated men of sickly health, miserable habits and more miserable propensities ...'[35] When the newly formed Medical Staff Corps was established in June 1855, FN's managerial and administrative expertise – as well as her important contacts back in England – may have kickstarted the organisation of this significant development, but as we can see, it is almost criminal it was not initiated when the problems were identified a few months earlier by Dr Smith.[36] This can also be said of Smith's recommendations derived from reports sent back from Constantinople by three of his officers. One of these, Dr Dumbreck, recommended two types of uniform for soldiers due to the extreme cold and hot climate, the risk of high fevers and dysentery due to the swampy marshland and unhygienic conditions. Dumbreck also advised the need for strict hygiene practices in the military camps and for fresh water, noting rather prophetically that, 'The air is surcharged with the elements of disease, and if we are deficient in supplies on which the maintenance of their stamina depends, we shall have much to contend with.' During March 1854, Smith also wrote to the military secretary with urgent recommendations for extra hospital marquees to avoid sick soldiers having to sleep on the ground, as well as sending out an extra 40,000 cholera belts (when it was believed flannel cloth around the abdomen would protect the stomach and bowels from the cold) and peat charcoal for disinfecting.[37] Needless to say, none of these early 1854 recommendations was acted upon.

Interestingly, as early as 1819, John Millingen wrote of the considerable roles needed to attend to general hospitals erected in the military field, and one can see the similarities to FN's request of a workable system from her letter to Sidney Herbert in January 1855; these were not new ideas. Roles such as a Steward of the Hospital, a principal Ward Master to each military division, a Porter in charge of gates and keys, a Principal Cook and various Store Keepers (medical equipment, arms etc) were all suggested. Next came the 'under-servants' to serve the previously mentioned roles; here we have orderlies working the wards, kitchen and mortuary, as well bathers to assist - you've guessed it – with baths. Then we have the statement that, 'The female attendants should be as few as possible and consist of 1) A Matron, 2) A Nurse to each division, 3) Washerwomen and sempstresses [sempster was a male tailor, also another term of seamstress], when washing must necessarily be performed within the precincts of the hospital.'[38] Nurses were to be accommodated separately wherever possible and concern themselves with preparing comforts from the kitchens (puddings and other 'delicate' foodstuffs) and be strictly forbidden for dealing with foul linen due to their handling of food. Such recommendations make sense, however, 'their personal attendance upon the sick is seldom if ever of any use and their presence in the wards ... is always a source of altercation and confusion both amongst the patients and the orderlies.'[39] Matrons however, in addition to superintending the female staff and reporting any 'irregularities', are stated as being

> ... of great economical importance; but to fulfil the expectations which such an appointment leads us to, it is absolutely requisite that she be selected in a class of women who would not conceive the many unpleasant duties attached to the station, as derogatory to their rank or painful to their feelings; a steady and well-behaved non-commissioned officer's wife or widow, should be the person generally preferred.[40]

The first recorded mentions of a military 'fixed' hospital (which became known as the general hospital) in March 1690 listed thirty nurses as part of a regular staff; these nurses were paid only 1 shilling less that a surgeon's mate and 2 shillings more than soldiers' wives who nursed/cooked/washed and were listed under 'servants', showing they must have had some training and were probably considered a professional nurse.[41] The fact FN's experimental role of taking female nurses directly to military hospitals and areas of war had to be approved by parliament with many regulations, show remnants of these early nineteenth century opinions on nursing still existed. One only has to look at the agreement drawn up by the War Office on 19 October 1854, where although FN was named 'Superintendent of the female nursing establishment in the English General Military Hospitals in Turkey', she also had instructions to communicate immediately on arrival to the Chief Medical Officer at Scutari. FN was to act only under his orders and direction when carrying out her duties. The letter also confirmed the allotment of nurses, and their duties were under FN's control but only under the approval and sanction of the Chief Medical Officer. Despite how the nursing experiment looked and sounded, it was not a case of any female nurse being in charge, not at the beginning anyway. A full transcript of the letter of engagement can be found in Sir Edward Cook's biography (Volume 1), pp.155-6.

We have already seen that the first small group of nursing nuns, the Sisters of Mercy, had left their Bermondsey Convent in the early hours of 17 October 1854 to make their way to Paris. After eventually finding a hotel to stay in, a telegram from Dr Grant arrived the next day instructing them to stay in Paris until further notice. This was given in the form of a letter on 19 October, informing the Sisters of Mercy that the government had finally organised an official nursing expedition, headed up by Florence Nightingale, and that they were to await the arrival of the newly formed nursing government party.

Recruiting suitable nurses had been difficult. FN, foreseeing problems in the women coming forward, such as lack of character, slovenly behaviour etc. (after all, she had had experience in this), had originally only wanted twenty nurses to be the upper limit to take with her. Sidney Herbert, however, had insisted on forty, with instructions to recruit across religions. Due to the anti-Irish feeling in the general public that we have already discussed, coupled with further political sensitivities, Herbert instructed FN to recruit Catholics, but not too many; in fact, one Catholic to ten Protestants would suffice. After all, the government did – and were – depending on Irish votes. Indeed, after much fervour over the few days FN had to arrange this unprecedented trip, she asked her friends Mrs Herbert, Mary Stanley and Selena Bracebridge to interview for nurses, which was duly conducted at the Herbert home in Belgrave Square, London. After much despair of the low quality of women who applied (who appeared to apply mainly for money, not from a place of empathic care) forty nurses were selected; sixteen hospital working-class nurses, ten Catholic nuns (five from the Sisters of Mercy convents in Bermondsey and five from the Convent of Our Lady of the Orphans in Norwood), eight Anglican Sisters and six from St John's House (a lay Sisterhood and one of the first nurse training schools in the country, established in 1848). FN took the only nurse she felt suitable from the Harley Street Clinic with her, which was Mrs Clarke, a Matron, although in this context, 'Matron' was more a housekeeper, not the senior nurse we would recognise today. In the end, thirty-eight nurses arrived at Constantinople in November 1854; one nurse having been dismissed before leaving London for being unsuitable and another from France due to illness. Both were hospital nurses. FN had departed for France on 21 October where she made an appointment to recruit more Catholic nuns from the famous Daughters of Charity, who, as we have already seen, had years of military nursing expertise. Despite this, the Order of St Vincent de Paul refused FN's request. Finally, on 23/24 October 1854, FN united with the nursing contingent led by her family friends, Selena and Charles Bracebridge, with the Bermondsey nuns waiting in Paris and on 25 October, the complete party continued their journey towards the Crimea.[42]

It was the next contingent of nurses sent out by the government that would lay the foundations for the fiery relationships encountered between FN, Betsy and Bridgeman. On 2 December 1854, Mary Stanley, Nightingale's good friend and one of those who had helped to recruit appropriate ladies for the Crimea, headed up a party of forty-seven volunteers including fifteen nuns belonging to the Sisters of Mercy, twenty-two hospital working-class nurses and nine Ladies (wealthy women that did not work and were deemed to have natural authority), who all left London enroute to do their bit for nursing in the Crimean War. It is well recorded in the contemporary sources that this venture was not welcome or wanted and went down like a lead balloon with FN. It is also the point of history where Betsy

Cadwaladyr and Mother Mary Francis Bridgeman enter the story. So, what went wrong?

Charles and Selina Bracebridge were friends of the Nightingale family and accompanied FN on her departure to the Crimea in October. Charles Bracebridge (1799 – 1872) was on a similar society level as FN's father and came from a wealthy merchant family. In 1824, he married Miss Selina Mills (1800 – 1874) who was a promising young artist and together they had interests in travel, writing and medical reform for the poor. It was Selina who had taken FN to a workhouse infirmary to see the horrors for herself. In 1847, FN became unwell with what was likely depression at her situation of not being able to follow her nursing dreams, and the Bracebridge's suggested to the Nightingale family that she travelled to Rome with them to recuperate. Selina became a second mother to FN, but one that recognised her needs to operate outside the societal norms of what was expected of her, especially from her immediate family.[43]

It was apparently a letter from Charles Bracebridge to Sidney Herbert, sent whilst in the Crimea, that started the ball rolling for a second party of nurses. A letter from Lady Charlotte Canning, who had helped interview nurses for FN and who chaired the committee for the Harley Street Clinic, to Lady Stratford, the wife of the Ambassador, who ended up assisting the new party on their arrival, states that 'Mr Bracebridge had distinctly asked for them [nurses] by letter as for any articles of any sort or kind and he always wrote for Miss Nightingale.'[44] This letter has not survived, if it ever existed, but two contemporary accounts of a letter being sent cannot be ignored. Fanny Taylor, one of the Lady Nurses in the second group, wrote in her book reflecting on her time in the Crimea:

> The medical men in England said the numbers of nurses already gone were but as a drop in the ocean amidst the thousands now in the Eastern hospitals; a second band was to be in readiness to go if sent for. The summons came in a letter from Mr. Bracebridge

to Mr. Herbert, who, anxious that as many as possible should benefit by the care of nurses, determined to send out as large a staff as were ready. With as much care as was possible, a selection was made from the registered candidates.[45]

It is interesting to note the words 'from the registered candidates', thus clarifying the immense response they had from women wishing to nurse in a war zone and who had continued to gather at the Herbert's home in Belgrave Square in the hope of being selected if another batch of nurses were sent. FN's sister, Parthenope, had written to their father complaining of so many having to be interviewed and notes the amount at one point being 307! Just over 600 applicant letters survive today and are kept at The National Archives.[46]

Consideration must be given to the fact that Herbert may have misread an innocent comment in the Bracebridge letter that more nurses maybe welcomed if needs be; a point suggested both by Bostridge in his biography of Nightingale in 2009 and by Helmstadter in her book on nursing in the Crimea in 2020. Bostridge goes onto say that added to that confusion may be the fact Mrs Herbert was 'overwhelmed in a sea of nurses' and suggested they were just waiting to see if Nightingale did NOT want any more nurses sent over.[47] Interestingly, in her journal on her Crimean experience, Bridgeman notes that after preparations were made for more Sisters of Mercy to go to the Crimea in this second batch of nurses, they had left Ireland for London on 3 November only to find much uncertainty. She noted that '… the delay on the part of the War Office was caused by doubt as to the reception Miss Nightingale, and her party, should receive from the medical and other authorities in the East; that until this could be ascertained, the War Office dared not send out an additional number.'[48] In whatever manner the letter may or may not have been interpreted, the second party of nurses arrived in Constantinople on 17 December 1854, only to be told they were not wanted or needed. Which, as one can imagine, did not go down very well. For the time being, however, we will concentrate on how this affected Mother Bridgeman and Betsy Cadwaladyr.

## Selection for nursing

The two main sources for Nightingale to take nurses with her were from the hospitals and from the Sisterhoods, who had long been tending to the needs of the sick poor in their communities, despite misgivings from Sidney Herbert due to the political Irish connotations. As well as sensitive and timed communication, it was a case of who you knew and where you knew them that enabled the Irish-English barrier to be broken down for the Irish nurses to do their bit for nursing in the Crimea. The Very Reverend Dr Henry Manning (who had converted from Anglicism to Catholicism in 1851), and who was intimate friends with the Herberts, Stanleys and the Nightingales, became the common link between religion, War Office and convent. He was keen to see the Catholic Sisters play their part.[49]

The Vicar General of Westminster, Dr Robert Whitty, advised the Vicar General of Dublin, Dr Yore, that the War Office had confirmed arrangements with the Bishop of Southwark to recruit Sisters of Mercy as nurses to send to the Crimea.[50] A Vicar General was a powerful position and these roles acted as a stand-in for the archbishop when he was away (in this case, Archbishop Wiseman was in Rome). Dr Robert Whitty just so happened to be the brother of Sister Mary Vincent Whitty, the Superioress of the Sisters of Mercy parent convent in Baggott Street, Dublin, and when shown the contents of his letter to Dr Yore, she immediately offered the services of the Sisters of Mercy. She in turn wrote to the Reverend Mothers asking them to send who they could to Baggott Street: 'The Government has virtually applied for Sisters, and offered to pay their expenses; and as there is no time to be lost, I beg of you to send your candidates on Tuesday or Wednesday, to St Catherine's [Baggot Street] and if their service be not required they can return.'[51] The response was immense. In the end, eleven Irish Sisters were selected and four from English convents. Two from the Carlow convent – Sister Mary Aloysius Doyle and Sister Mary Stanislaus (Heyfron) – were selected due to their youth, good health and experience in nursing in a recent cholera outbreak; Doyle's journal is only one of three to have survived and provides a wonderful insight to her experiences.[52]

Mother Mary Vincent Whitty and Bridgeman travelled ahead to London and on 4 November 1854, the day that FN arrived in Constantinople, both Sisters of Mercy met Sidney Herbert at his home in Belgrave Square. Here, he explained there would be a slight delay in sending the nursing party over to the Crimea as he needed to hear from FN in Scutari first. He also agreed to a priest travelling with them, but not as their chaplain due to arousing negative connotations from the world of politics. This went against their initial agreement arranged by Dr Grant with the War Office: 'Fifth – that there shall always be a priest to provide for the spiritual care of the Sisters, and that the War Office authorities would attach to the hospital, with this view, the priest who should be selected as most fit for the assistance of the Sisters.'[53] Sidney Herbert later reneged on this, saying that any priest chosen by the Catholic superiors could not travel with the Sisters and there was to be no discussion on this.

During this time in London, Bridgeman gained some knowledge of hospital nursing by going to St George's Hospital, as well as others, in London, and notes that despite being in religious dress, the Sisters were civilly treated by all. Their priest, Father Ronan, had been approved by Dr Manning in November 1854 and would eventually come to join Bridgeman and her Sisters on 21 January 1855, being discharged home on 2 September 1855 after an illness.[54] Bridgeman was unanimously elected as Mother Superior for the group for the entirety of their time in the Crimea, this was confirmed by Dr Yore on 24 November and agreed by the War Office.[55] However, as well as the delay in waiting to see if FN wanted more nurses sent over, there was also the issue of Sidney Herbert retracting his promise to the Sisters that a chaplain for their spiritual needs could travel with them. On the eve of departure, they were given the following ultimatum: abort the mission or travel without a priest. Bridgeman was not stupid enough to believe aborting would help their cause and thus agreed to go ahead and rely on God '... who has never forsaken us or failed to raise up for us friends in the hour of need'.[56] Finally, on 2 December 1854, the party of fifteen nuns, twenty-two hospital nurses (including Betsy) and ten Ladies (including the Superintendent of the party, Mary Stanley) left London for France, enroute to the Crimea.

Betsy comes across as more pragmatic in her autobiographical account of being selected for the second party of nurses under Mary Stanley. We saw in Chapter 4 how Betsy had been staying with her sister, Bridget, in London when she had read the historic report in *The Times* regarding the state of the soldiers in the Crimea and the herculean effort of FN and the War Office to take nurses into a war zone. It was at this stage Betsy announced – a statement that is often repeated when examining this part of the Crimean history – that, 'I read of Miss Nightingale preparing to take out nurses. I did not like the name of Nightingale. When I first hear a name, I am very apt to know by my feeling whether I shall like the person who bears it.'[57] Her biographer, Jane Williams, adds a footnote to this: 'The peculiar tone of the heroine's mind is strongly marked by the premonitory [something bad before it happens] form of prejudice against a name which conveys to people in general a very pleasing impression.' This is a hint of the strained relationship that Betsy and FN initially enjoyed in the Crimea, although this must be balanced with FN's comments when Betsy had to be invalided home on 3 November 1855: 'Sent home Novr 3 /55 in the *Cleopatria* on account of ill health. Parted with the greatest regret & recommended for a twelve months wages.' This shows how much FN recognised and appreciated Betsy's part in the nursing experiment of the Crimea.[58]

Betsy was initially informed by the solicitor named in the newspaper article requesting nurses to go to the Crimea that she was three days too late to leave with the first party.[59] Undeterred, she obtained a recommendation from a Dr Watkins, an old acquaintance from Wales. On the register of *Nurses sent to the Military Hospitals in the East*, we can see Betsy had – in addition to the recommendation from Dr Watkins – a reference from none other than Lady Llanover, stating Betsy was 'well known and respected by Lady Hall of

Llanover'. Interestingly, the Register entry gives Betsy the age of 55, although she was actually 65 at this point; the chances are she would have been flatly refused by the authorities if her true age was known. Although interviewed by Mary Stanley, she was told there was little hope of being selected and there were no more nurses to be sent out until, or even if, FN requested them. However, a couple of days later, a message arrived from Liz Herbert asking Betsy to attend the Herbert residence that same day between 10am and 12pm; according to Betsy, it was already 2pm when she received the message, but she still set out and was told she was not too late, whereby a clothing fitting began for Betsy's mission to the Crimea. She was accepted into Stanley's second party of nurses, thanks probably in no large coincidence to the connection with Lady Llanover and the fact she did not fit the Sarah Gamp parody so feared at this time.[60]

After a rough journey from Folkestone to Boulogne, a stay over in Paris and then the steamer boat being grounded at Lyons for two hours, the travelling party missed their train to Marseilles. After much fussing around, this second party of Crimean nurses managed to catch a later train, but the sea-crossing from Marseilles to Constantinople was also fraught with difficulties, beginning with the state of their boat, the *Egyptus*. Due to a shortage of troop ships, this old mailboat had been used to ferry between 200 and 300 French soldiers at the time of Stanley's party boarding on the 7 December. According to Fanny Taylor in her book on her experiences in the Crimea, the *Egyptus* should have been back in the dock six months earlier for repair, with decks that needed caulking and 'nothing being secure'.[61] Betsy, an experienced sailor with years of travel under her belt, noted that the mailboat was 'a perfect rolling pin' and that although the *Egyptus* should have been in the docks for repair, the 'fault was in her building'.[62] To top it all off, there were no first-class berths for the Sisters of Mercy as they were all allocated to the Ladies; something that horrified Bridgeman. In a sweeping statement of snobbery, she noted in her diary that this '… represented the evil consequences of being thrown thus into domestic contact with this class of people'.[63]

Although Mary Stanley and Fanny Taylor tried to assist, they could only obtain berths for a few of the nuns, something Bridgeman declined as she wished to keep the Sisters all together. Shortly after departure, a ferocious storm sent the boat into the port of Hyeres, about 55 miles along the southern French coast. The gales died down by the afternoon and the ship commenced its journey on the evening of 8 December. Bridgeman notes how, when sitting down for their first dinner that a '… crowd of coarse men rushed in and sat down without ceremony' causing Bridgeman to gather her Sisters – without eating – to their sleeping quarters, whereafter on the voyage, one of the couriers travelling with them, Angelo, made sure the Sisters of Mercy ate their dinner earlier, in private.[64]

However, bad weather continued to plague the voyage. On 12 December, Stanley's party were caught in yet another storm, this one causing many to think they would die. Bridgeman notes that the top of their cabin was blown off and water descended into their quarters. Sister Aloysius Doyle also noted the top of their cabin was blown away, and that the boat tilted to one side as waves crashed against it relentlessly, to the point where she thought each wave would be their last.[65] Fanny Taylor wrote that the cabins the nurses and nuns occupied were the worst affected:

> The scene of the storm was past description; the men darted in to bail out the water; some of the nurses were too sick to care for anything … and others began to prepare for instant death. Sisters and nurses were to be seen, ankle deep in water, assisting the bare-legged sailors to bail out their cabins, in which were floating oranges, books, clothes, &c. When daylight came, the poor sisters found that the sea had penetrated into their trunks; and books and clothes, and ornaments for their chapel, were entirely spoiled. The misery the poor sisters endured, and most patiently, during this voyage, baffles description. No breakfast could be got that day; so sick and well fasted till dinner time, when the storm began to abate.[66]

Bridgeman was noted for her calmness and unwavering faith during the storm, although it is interesting to note that Betsy does not dwell on this episode in her autobiography, with the exception of 'We had a troublesome voyage'.[67] Perhaps, with all her past worldly travels, Betsy had experienced such storms before. However, there is a supplement to this particular episode, written by someone only identified as a fellow voyager with hospital experience and a probationer at St John's House. We know that after the first group of nurses went out with FN, the London committee of ladies who interviewed and selected the nurses then insisted any further recruits would need to spend time in a London hospital for clinical experience, with St John's House being one of those who agreed to board the ladies during this time as short-term probationers.[68] The anonymous writer then goes into more detail, confirming the suffering of the occupants of the forward cabins which housed the nuns and the nurses; screaming could be heard and with each crashing wave it was assumed the boat would sink and death would come soon.[69]

After the journey they had all been through, it is easy to understand the frustration, anger and shock felt by Stanley's party on arrival at Constantinople on 17 December after being told they were 'Not wanted at Scutari, the War Office made a mistake in sending out the party. No room for them…' and that there was no accommodation or employment for them. FN had communicated to Lord Stratford Canning, the British Ambassador staying at Therapia, that she must '… at once ask your Excellency to provide for the reception, lodging, and maintenance of this party, which may arrive without further notice'.[70] None of them could understand at this point how FN's outburst was likely borne from frustration and the difficulties of not only controlling their deployment and their behaviour, but that she was also still trying to smooth the communication and working relationships with the medical officers. Whilst trying to look outside of the Scutari hospital for them, FN mentions in a letter to Sidney Herbert on Christmas Day 1854 that the medical officers of the convalescent hospitals, the Merchant Seaman's hospital, had declined her offer of female nurses. Neither Bridgeman nor Besty would have understood the political pressures that FN was under, as well as her own life's mission to make nursing more respectable.[71]

Betsy recalls that she '… was very much disappointed, like the rest of Miss Stanley's party, at being sent to Therapia, instead of having employment at once in some military hospital … I was discontented and uncomfortable.' While Bridgeman states, 'This was an indescribable shock to us all'. After docking at Constantinople on the afternoon of 17 December 1854, a messenger was sent to FN at the Scutari hospital to announce the Stanley party's arrival, but that evening, it was Charles Bracebridge who returned to the party to announce that a small boat would arrive in the morning to convey them to Therapia, the summer residence of the British Embassy, which they duly did late the next morning.[72] Except, however, for Bridgeman and her Sisters of Mercy. In her journal, Bridgeman states that after discussion with Mary Stanley, a request was made for hospitality from the Sisters of Charity at nearby Galata for approximately a week, when it was hoped this delay would be sorted. The joy at being in a convent and praying again was a balm to the Sisters of Mercy, but according to Bridgeman, they soon discovered that the Sisters of Charity had had to cancel their 'pension school' (a form of private education for wealthier Catholic families) to make room for Bridgeman and her Sisters to eat and sleep.[73] However, Fanny Taylor notes that the Sisters of Charity sent the offer as their boarding school had closed and thus had room to accommodate the fifteen Sisters of Mercy for a short time. Sister Aloysius Doyle also writes that a message sent from Bridgeman to the Sisters of Charity was received well and they '… were shown into a large schoolroom that had just been emptied of school children to accommodate us'.[74]

Meanwhile, Betsy and the rest of Stanley's party duly made their way to the summer residence of the British Embassy at Therapia, a village approximately 15 miles further up the Bosphorus and now part of modern-day Istanbul. Therapia, meaning cure/healing of the sick and seen today in the words therapy/therapeutic, was described as a Greek village by Miss Fanny Taylor in her account on her time nursing in the Crimea. It was also home to a naval hospital that had first been established there in January 1854, two months before the war officially broke out. The navy up to this point had a history of a better standard of healthcare, with mortality falling 'from 1:8 in 1780 to 1:30 in 1812'[75] and the service has been much overlooked during the Crimea due to the army hospitals and their Nightingale nursing experiment. By the start of the Crimea, the navy had a better supply of medicinal equipment, medicines and comforts for the sick and, due to a better organised administrative system, fresh food and drink was easily supplied to war ships via naval onshore hospitals.[76]

Therapia was described as being

> a large wooden, rickety three-storied, Turkish private house situated ten feet from the banks of the Bosphorus and standing only three feet above water level. When taken over, the first floor was arranged as wards for sixty patients; wash-houses and storerooms were on the ground floor. An adjoining building afforded accommodation for thirty officers and in yet another building the kitchen was installed. The whole was surrounded by a walled enclosure and from the windows of the wards the gay and beautiful Bosphorus was to be seen.[77]

Dr John Davidson was the medical director and was fully aware of the lack of skilled nurses; he and his immediate superior, Dr David Deas, finally convinced the Board of Admiralty to find suitable female nurses. On the 10 January 1855, Therapia saw the arrival of Eliza McKenzie with a small party of nurses and her husband, the Reverand John McKenzie, younger son of the 7th Baronet of Coul, a scientist. Eliza, meanwhile, was the daughter of Thomas Chalmers, the founder of the Scottish Free Church. Eliza became a valuable asset, managing her nurses well (three Ladies and three professional nurses) and even earning a very rare accolade of being made an honorary member of the Officer's Mess. Eliza herself was a trained nurse, having worked in the Middlesex Hospital and after successfully managing the Naval Therapia Hospital, she returned home in November 1855 after suffering exhaustion.[78]

It is possible that Eliza McKenzie may have met Betsy, as shortly before Eliza's arrival at Therapia, the surgeons asked Stanley's nurses if they would help with the washing of three months' worth of linen whilst the hospital awaited the arrival of Eliza and her nurses. Stanley placed one of the Lady Volunteers, whom Betsy names as Miss Shaw Stewart, in charge of a rota of the paid nurses, not all of whom were happy. Betsy gladly took her turn in this rota: 'With her [Stanley's] permission, I took my turn among the nurses who went up to the naval hospital to wash clothes for the patients. I was glad to do anything that was of use to the poor fellows.'[79] The nurses also helped the naval hospital not only with washing but also sewing the linens, writing letters and caring for the sailors themselves on a weekly basis. When a few of Stanley's party became unwell, the naval surgeons tended to their medical needs.[80]

However, the sense of frustration and boredom that arose from waiting at Therapia is obvious in Betsy's account, as well as her utmost respect for Mary Stanley. Betsy was critical of some of the working-class nurses, stating many of them '... had never filled any place of trust before ... incapable of the duties which they had undertaken' whilst others were 'good women and excellent nurses.' Betsy continues to be somewhat more critical, noting the fellow nurses' 'ill-behaviour' and blaming alcohol for at least the behaviour of a few of the women. However, Betsy also empathises with the fact they had all left their homes and families to – how they saw it – sit around and wait when they knew soldiers needed their help.[81] Her full sympathies lay firmly with Mary Stanley and her task in finding them all work, as well as coping with the behaviour of some of the women, calling her a 'proper lady' and noting her calmness and patience despite the stress she was under. Betsy disapproved of the way the women flocked around Stanley when she returned to them and acknowledges that some of the women sniped and blamed Stanley for the situation they were in. Betsy's narrative shows her as one of the party eager to get stuck in, so to speak, but also remaining separate from the drunkenly disorder of some of the group and being able to see the bigger picture of the situation they found themselves in.

Betsy's account is echoed in the narrative of Fanny Taylor. She, too, admired Stanley's patience and hard work in securing them all a place in the nursing roles they had all signed up for. Taylor is also aware of the travelling Mary Stanley had to do, from the British Embassy nearby in Pera to Scutari itself and makes note of their anxieties awaiting Stanley's return. When she did return, many of the nurses became irritated with her 'vagueness' and that there was no answer given for their delay in getting to nurse the soldiers. However, Taylor also notes that Stanley was '… beloved by all for her just government of the community, her uniform sweetness of temper, and thoughtful kindness for all'. Yet some irritation can be felt by Taylor's further narrative:

> Wherever the fault lay, it was most unaccountable that 47 women should be kept idle at Therapia, while so much work was to be done at Scutari—when the hospitals were crowded, and the numbers [of death and disease] greater than at any previous period ... If there were really no room to be found for us at the Hospital, why were we not accommodated with a house in Scutari? There could have been no difficulty in this, for houses in Scutari were procured for other purposes. But there were many strange things done at this period, and no doubt many others strangely left undone. If we had been only allowed to help in the cooking—there were but 12 cooks for upwards of 3,000 sick—it would no doubt have promoted the well-being, and alleviated much of the sufferings, of the poor patients.[82]

Shortly, Betsy would indeed be one of the much-needed cooks.

Bridgeman was also known for her patience during the wait for work. Sister Doyle notes that after Christmas 1854, the Sisters were longing to work and that after hearing hundreds were dying every month, as noted by Taylor above, they felt they were wasting time. Bridgeman would calmly reassure her group until the day when, finally, an initial five nuns – including Bridgeman – were asked to go to Scutari General hospital.[83]

The routine of feeding patients was of great concern to FN. In one of her many letters to Sidney Herbert, dated 8 January 1855, she states that food should be cooked by cooks, not drunken soldiers and that orderlies are often ill and not wanted by their regiments. Then on 28 January, she wrote that the drawing and serving of food to patients was useless and 'extra diet' kitchens should be established to serve arrow root and beef tea, staples of nutrition for the injured troops.[84]

The healing effect of properly prepped and served food had been noticed – albeit anecdotally – by one of the nursing sisters who had gone out to the Crimea with FN originally. Sister Anne Terrot, one of the Sellonites, worked on a ward at Scuatri with her fellow nurse, Sister Elizabeth. They were assigned to different medical officers, with Sister Elizabeth assigned to one – Dr Maclean – who took his time with the patients and prescribed more extras such as wine, milk and pudding. The other (unnamed) officer Terrot worked with, did not:

> There was a great difference in the amount of extras we distributed, and I soon observed a corresponding difference in the number of deaths, and was convinced that the careful feeding up system they pursued did preserve or at least prolong life ... I forget the exact proportion, but I think at the end of a week the deaths in my wards nearly doubled hers, while there was no such difference in the nature of the cases as to account for it. Indeed, the most hopeless cases seemed to be given to

Maclean, and the only cause I could see for his losing fewer patients seemed to be his very careful feeding-up system and his careful medical treatment.[85]

A large part of the nurses' work and duties was firstly related to diet and then laundry. When the female nurses began arriving at the Crimean military hospitals, they found any type of cooking and facilities were horrendously defective, the standard of food left wanting and dietary needs for the sick – such as beef tea and arrow root – rarely supplied.[86] The need for an adequate diet in illness and recovery has long been recognised; the ancients advised following a seasonal diet to complement and/or rectify the imbalances of the four humours and medieval medicine, especially on the medieval battlefield, knowledge of diet to aid recovery was as important as pain relief.[87] Military hospitals at this point in the Crimea had a regime of various diets, with a full diet consisting of 1 pound of meat, 1 pound of potatoes, 2 pints of tea and half a pint of porter (a type of beer); half diet and low diet were half and quarter of the full amount. A spoon diet consisted of half a pound of bread and tea and was for those who were gravely ill and in the care of the nurses. The surgeon could prescribe 'diet extras' such as beef tea, arrow root, rice, fowl, mutton, milk, sago (plant starch) and lemons/sugar for lemonade, hence FN introducing 'extra diet kitchens' and an area of work that Betsy became the head of at Balaklava hospital. In fact, recorded deaths for one regiment, the 4th Light Dragoons, dropped from seventy-eight to thirty-three by January 1855, with warmer clothing and more meat being supplied to the men stated as the reason.[88] However, Taylor notes in her book that although the food sounded and would indeed be amply sufficient back home in England, in Turkey the meat especially was 'wretchedly inferior'.[89] Malnutrition was rife. And it was this report of 'near-starvation' reported in *The Times* that the celebrated Victorian chef, the French-born Alexis Soyer, favourite of the rich and famous, came to offer his services to the War Office in February 1855.

## Alexis Soyer

Soyer had a fundamental and honed understanding of nutrition developed over the years and had assisted with recipes in the Irish Famine of 1847. In January 1855, a letter from a soldier serving in the Crimean War was printed in *The Times* asking him to suggest a recipe or two with only a dearth of rations and fuel available to them in the field, as well as a general lack of knowledge and cooking skills. This he did by experimenting with the requests and developing *Soyer's Camp Receipts for the Army in the East*. His previous publications *Soyer's Shilling Cookery* and *The Modern Housewife* were already being used amongst the soldiers in the Crimea in an attempt to help their deprived rations more palatable. His offer to develop a field stove to use at Scutari and then to implement that model, if successful, to other hospitals, was quickly approved and his efforts greatly improved things in the war zones.[90] Tea, for example, a greatly prescribed item, was usually tied in a cloth and made in the same boilers and cauldrons as the meat; the cloth shrunk with tea inside and sunk to the bottom. Even Fanny Taylor makes mention of the tea being 'the most wretched stuff possible'.[91] Soyer quite rightly said the tea needed to be diffused in the water instead of just sitting at the bottom in a heap so, using a coffee filter, he made the 'Scutari Teapot', with one teapot amount based on twenty men. The result was that only four teapots were needed for one hospital as each teapot made a quarter more tea than expected, and made a clear, sediment-free tea which was quickly approved by FN.[92]

Soyer's other resounding success was his field kitchen stove, enabling the men battling nature as much as the enemy to have proper cooked, more nutritious food. With a model based on that one letter from a soldier in January 1855, Soyer describes his Field Stove thus:

> Each stove will consume not more than from 12 to 15lbs. of fuel, and allowing 20 stoves to a regiment, the consumption would be 300lbs. per thousand men. The allowance per man is, I believe,

3.5lbs each, which gives a total of 3500lbs. per thousand men. The economy of fuel would consequently be 3200lbs. per regiment daily. Coal will burn with the same advantage. Salt beef, pork, Irish stew, stewed beef tea, coffee, cocoa etc, can be prepared in these stoves and with the same economy. They can also be fitted with an apparatus for baking, roasting, and steaming.[93]

This is confirmed by letters from those in the field, as seen below, and from FN herself:

Head-Quarters, Sebastopol, 19th *June*, 1856.

Sir,
In acknowledging your letter of the 15th instant, I have to observe that one of your camp-stoves has been in constant use in the 56th Regiment for the last two months, and from inquiries from the men themselves, and by my own observation, I am decidedly of opinion that they possess very considerable advantages over any other means of cooking at present in the use in the British army, and I would strongly advocate their being furnished to all barracks, not only on account of their superiority in rendering the soldiers' rations much more wholesome than when prepared by the means ordinarily used, but also for their great economy of fuel and labour. All these advantages were clearly demonstrated on the occasion of Lord Gough's [aide-de-camp to Lord Raglan] visit to the camp of the 56th when, with ten of the stoves in operation, you superintended so successfully the cooking of five hundred men's rations.
     I remain, your very obedient servant, A. W. Lacy,
      Lieut-Col., *commanding* 56th *regiment.*[94]

FN noted that 'Soyer's Stoves will boil, stew, bake and steam, in short; do everything but grill; ensuring that variety in cooking which is proved essential to health ... and found most useful in the Crimea.'[95]

Interestingly, in May1855, Soyer and Betsy met in the extra diet kitchen at Balaklava General hospital, with Soyer heaping praise on Betsy. FN, feeling at this point that the hospital in Scutari was running better, made her first trip to the Crimean war front with Mrs Roberts, FN's aide-de-camp, and three other nurses, while Charles Bracebridge and Soyer joined them to visit the military kitchens. Miss Weare, the superintendent of nursing at the Balaklava General hospital at this time was giving them a guided tour. Soyer was impressed in what Betsy could manage to cook with little ingredients and equipment, making a note for new utensils and advising recipes to her and, in Soyer's words - ' ... then we left Miss Davis, much pleased with Miss Nightingale's kind remarks, my approbation of her services, and, above all, very proud of having, two days before, been visited and highly complimented by Lady Stratford de Redcliffe and the other ladies.'[96] Betsy notes in her autobiography of her admiration of Lady Stratford; on this occasion, a brief visit to her extra diet kitchen is mentioned and crossing words with FN, where she told her, a tad sarcastically, that she might as well have expected the queen. Betsy did not mention Soyer, or his praises of her, and if he seemed to think Betsy was overjoyed at their praises of her work, she most certainly was not overjoyed enough to write about it![97]

## Balaklava

In January 1855, Lord Raglan had requested eight nurses to help on the war front in the Crimea in the Balaklava General hospital and Lord Stratford planned on opening up extra beds at Koulali. This month was becoming the worst for mortality than even Dr Andrew Smith or FN could have imagined; the death rate was over 60 per cent, averaging forty-five deaths a day, mainly from dysentery/bowel issues as well as fever. Sister Anne Terot notes how 'It seemed a common occurrence in this corridor and the adjoining wards for a man to be found dead, neither orderly nor patient in the next bed being aware of it'.[98] However, the news of opportunities in a hospital caused some excitement amongst Mary Stanley's nurses at finally having a purpose for which they had volunteered.

On 6 January 1855, whilst still at Therapia, Bridgeman received an unexpected visit from Mother Mary Moore, the Reverend Mother Superior of the original five members of the Sisters of Mercy from the Bermondsey Convent in London, who had travelled with FN in October 1854. She oversaw the extra diet kitchen at Scutari Barrack Hospital and – unlike Bridgeman – had a good working relationship with FN. Moore also earned much respect from the army due to her excellent management skills. Moore expressed FN's wishes that Bridgeman would be one of the five nuns of whom FN and Bridgeman had recently been communicating about, via letter since Christmas, to move to Scutari General hospital, about a mile away from the Scutari Barrack Hospital. However, this would not be to nurse, but rather to work in stores or the kitchens as there had been a lull in the war and there were no injured or wounded to currently take care of.

Needless to say, Bridgeman was not impressed with this as she was aware that the hospitals were full of men dying from cholera and dysentery. However, after agreeing to work under Moore with the proviso that Bridgeman could remove her nuns as and when she deemed fit, and until all Bridgeman's nuns could be reunited to work together again, Bridgeman and her four nuns arrived at Scutari General hospital on the 8 January 1855. Despite all five being extremely experienced nurses, especially when dealing with cholera, two Sisters (Agnes and Winifred) were immediately set to work in the kitchens under Moore; Sisters Aloysius Doyle and Elizabeth sorted linen and managed one of FN's stores, leaving Bridgeman to 'ladle soup'.[99] As one can imagine, this was not satisfactory to Bridgeman, who felt their time was wasted and her frustration can be felt in her journal:

Oh, the misery of that time; to sit in that one room without occupation; with a place to withdraw, even for a few moments, to seek recollection or to ask the aid and light we needed so much and then to know that we were surrounded by thousands of sufferers whom we had come so far and endured so many difficulties to serve.[100]

It was around this time that Betsy left for Scutari Barrack Hospital. In her autobiography, she shows some empathy for the Ladies Committee in London who, in her eyes, had shown a lack of knowledge of the working classes whilst recruiting. She felt women were sent out who were incapable of the duties and had never held positions of trust before, whereas others were excellent nurses and, above all, good and trustworthy women.[101] Betsy considered herself one of the latter and notes that after arriving at the Scutari Barrack Hospital, she was ready to work but nothing was given to them to do until the next day. And much to Betsy's chagrin, that work was in the linen stores. After a few days, and hearing of the request for nurses at Balaklava, Betsy demanded to be sent to the Crimea, the war front. She spoke first to Selina Bracebridge, who initially said there was no room, to which Betsy retaliated that there were 1,100-1,300 men in the hospital, and no one could know what Betsy could do whilst she just dealt with linen. Betsy also threatened to tell the country, via the newspapers, why she had returned home. Consequently, Selina Bracebridge arranged for FN to speak to Betsy and, as Betsy notes, this was the first time she had met FN.

Her 'Welsh blood was put up' when, aware and proud of her own faith and good behaviour, FN accused Betsy of upsetting other nurses and, if she did go to Balaklava, would be sent home if she misbehaved in any way. She was, after all, also going against FN's wishes. Betsy venomously denied upsetting anyone and had never been accused of misbehaving, stating simply that if she could not go the to hospital on the front lines at Balaklava, she would go home. Betsy describes FN in the most wonderful detail and although it cannot be corroborated by anyone else, it does seem typical of FN's frustrated reaction to something she could not control, while at the same time also showing her good side: "'If you go," she [FN] added, joining her open hands sideways together, and then forcibly dividing them, and spreading out her arms by her sides, "I have done with you and your new superintendent *entirely.*'" However, as that was Betsy's wish, FN then promised to get her on the next ship which could possibly be sailing the next day. Betsy does not elaborate how she knew the numbers of the men suffering in Balaklava, but a mere ten days later, she left on the ship *Melbourne* which, although meant to collect the eight nurses requested by Lord Raglan on 15 January, finally sailed on the 19th for the Crimea and the military hospital situated in the theatre of war, something neither Sidney Herbert nor FN had foreseen.[102]

We are lucky enough to have some finer details of the other seven nurses who accompanied Betsy to the Balaclava General hospital, all arriving on 23 January 1855. Emma Langston, one of the Church of England Sellonite Sisters, was made the Superintendent of Nursing by FN (although FN had no authority over the Crimean hospitals at this point). Two Ladies accompanied her, Martha Clough and Jane Shaw-Stewart from Therapia. As well as Betsy, the other four working-class nurses were Mrs Gibson, Mrs Whitehead, Mrs Mary Ann Noble and Mrs Disney. Mrs Jane Gibson was dismissed for intoxication and theft, so noted Selina Bracebridge, who was known for her harshness and what today might be called complete snobbery when looking down on the working class. In fact, on one occasion she noted a nurse was dismissed for inappropriate behaviour, which was then crossed out and corrected by Mary Stanley, who stated the nurse was sent home due to her health and that Bracebridge had never met her. Mrs Whitehead was a nurse who, according to Betsy, liked her drink, which was the cause of Whitehead breaking her leg and being laid up for a few months. She was then sent home by FN in October 1855 as her '… levity of conduct as to incapacitate her for work in the Hospital'. However, she was also described as a valuable nurse and recommended to receive two months' wages on her departure. Mrs Noble was invalided home due to broken health in July 1855, with FN recommending she have a year's wage from the War Office due to Mrs Noble being one of her best surgical nurses. Betsy herself was invalided home on 3 November 1855 due to ill health and the register notes how she was sent home with 'greatest regret' and recommended for a year's wages, even though FN would have liked to have kept her on until the end of the war.[103] This shows how FN appreciated Betsy's hard work in the extra diet kitchens.

On 21 January 1855 the arrival of Father William Ronan, a Catholic war chaplain and guardian to the Sisters of Mercy, arrived at the Scutari hospital to find the unacceptable circumstances to which the Sisters were keeping. After consultation with the Bishop of Constantinople, Father Ronan reiterated certain conditions for the Sisters, based upon their original conditions for going to the Crimea in the first place. These conditions included that all fifteen Sisters remain under the direction of Bridgeman, and that ten of the fifteen were to be sent to the Koulali hospital and the remaining five to be kept at either the Scutari Barrack or the Scutari General hospital, but that their community remained as one under Bridgeman. He also reiterated that they should have space to perform their religious needs and as they had pledged not to interfere with Protestant religion, they must be allowed to attend to the instruction and relief of all Catholics. Although Mother Mary Moore refused his guardianship, Father Ronan met with FN regarding Bridgeman's party. During his meeting with FN, he noted that should these conditions not be met, he had no choice but to remove them and return home.[104] FN agreed to the above and besides, Sidney Herbert did not want them to return home, especially for political reasons.

On 12 January 1855, Herbert wrote a letter to Bridgeman in which he apologised for their unexpected arrival in the Crimea and the reception they had received. Although he confirmed that FN had full authority, he felt his eagerness to accept offers of help, coupled with his misunderstanding of FN's nursing needs, had added to the Sisters of Mercy not being employed in the work they had hoped for. However, a post-script to this letter read: 'P.S. I am informed here that your kind services may very possibly be required at Galata which if it relieves you from your present difficulties, I should be glad to hear had been the case.' This turned out to be Koulali hospital, a Turkish barracks that had previously held Russian prisoners and was approximately 3 miles from Scutari. On 25 January 1855, Bridgeman and Sister Aloysius Doyle returned to Therapia to prepare to leave for Koulali with the remaining Irish Sisters of Mercy; Bridgeman had arranged replacements for herself and Doyle so five Sisters – Elizabeth Hersey, Clare Keane, Paula Rice, Winifred Sprey and Agnes Whitty – remained at Scutari General hospital. FN bid them a friendly and polite farewell after approving the plans. On 28 January, FN wrote a long letter to Sidney Herbert and mentioned the allocation of all the nurses: '19 have, at different times, gone home; 8 to Balaklava who I hope will come back for it is a mistake; 16 to Koulalee; 41 here [Scutari Barrack hospital]'.[105]

Bridgeman and her remaining nine Sisters arrived at Koulali in the afternoon of 27 January 1855 amongst a party of two ladies and four nurses under Mary Stanley as Superintendent. They had all been allocated five small rooms, uncleaned but whitewashed, recently occupied by patients, with a small kitchen and with a meagre food supply that was so bad, Bridgeman reports two of her Sisters falling ill. They found filthy wards and no kitchen or cooking facilities except large boilers in the Turkish cookhouse that needed a ladder to get to the hot water, which was then ladled out. This had a detrimental effect on the orderlies preparing arrowroot diets for the patients; the orderlies either served it uncooked and thus inedible, or not at all. The next day Mary Stanley had a meeting with the Principal Medical Officer at that time, Dr Nicholas O'Connor, who informed her that Koulali currently had around 500 patients and five doctors; he would like two nurses working with each doctor and the remainder would work in a nearby second Koulali hospital, known as the General Hospital, that was due to open for patients in the next couple of days. Stanley was also informed that it was the medical cases – fever, frostbite and diarrhoea were the main issues – not the surgical cases (as they now had the medical dressers for that), with which the nurses needed to be assisting, such as feeding patients appropriately and watching/monitoring them in a way that doctors could not. Bridgeman and her Sisters were given two rooms at the Koulali General hospital when it opened at the beginning of February and although she wrote about good relationships here with the medical men and the Ladies, she was glad to be away from the secular party. On the first day, Koulali General admitted approximately 200 soldiers and some of the nurses from Koulali Barracks hospital were sent to help, spending time washing, cutting the soldiers' hair, getting orderlies to dress the patients in clean shirts and feeding them the staple diet of arrowroot. All with too few beds and without a kitchen range, instead, wood fires and cauldrons were used.[106]

We do have a small amount of information on Dr Nicholas O'Connor, the Staff Surgeon in charge at Koulali when the nursing party arrived at the end of January 1855. He had gone to Scutari originally, in October 1854, but later died at Balaklava on 7 June 1856 and is buried at Balaklava Heights cemetery. His gravestone reads 'erected by his officer brothers' and, according to Shepherd in his *Crimean Doctors,* O'Connor is the only recorded suicide of a Crimean doctor, but unfortunately does not state his reference. O'Connor appears in another source as dying from 'disease', but on the Crimean hospital returns information from the government, suicide is listed under the heading 'disease'.[107]

Whilst all this allocation of nurses was going on, the hospitals were collapsing under the sheer volume of soldiers and their diseases and wounds. To give some idea of what Bridgeman and her Sisters were walking into at Koulali, and the mountain of administration that FN was tackling, bear in mind that the number of available beds across the Scutari and Koulali hospitals in January 1855 was just under 4,500, the largest being the Scutari Barrack hospital at 1,704 beds, where FN was stationed. For the Scutari and Koulali hospitals, in January 1855 alone (figures combined as Koulali had just opened in January 1855), there were 4,761 men admitted of which 1,393 (29 per cent) died. The highest cause of death in January was diarrhoea, with 841 men dying out of 1,480 admitted, including dysentery and colic; the second highest cause was fever, with 152 men dying out of 704 admitted, including typhus; thirdly, chronic and acute rheumatism, with forty-three men dying out of 596 admitted (see Appendix 2). In comparison, wounds and injuries accounted for only 228 admittances, of which 49 died.[108] Out of an overall total of 4,761 admitted in January alone, 2,877 (60 per cent) came from the Crimean war front. Of those 2,877 being transported, 239 (8 per cent) died during transportation. It is not difficult to see why men were found in corridors and were dying pitifully for want of proper nursing care and the need for proper, communicative transport.[109]

The overcrowding was borne out in Fanny Taylor's narrative on her first few days at Scutari Barrack hospital:

> All the corridors were thickly lined with beds, laid on low tressels [sic], raised a few inches from the ground. In the wards a divan runs round the room, and on this were laid the straw beds, and the sufferers on them. The hospital was crowded to its fullest extent. The building, which has since been reckoned to hold, with comfort, seventeen hundred men, then held nearly three thousand.[110]

Regarding transporting the ill and dying, Sister Terrot wrote that the

> sea itself became the grave of thousands. Sometimes on account of the Hospitals being full, and of the difficulties in landing, these sad cargoes lay on board ship for days after reaching Scutari; of course, numbers being daily thrown overboard, and thus lessening the difficulty in accommodating those who survived. Seeing the state of filth and neglect these poor men were in when landed, hearing how often they had implored in vain for a cup of water ... made me long for some organised

plan for supplying the transports with female nurses, but at that time it was impossible.[111]

Meanwhile, Besty was across the Black Sea at Balaklava. On 10 January 1855, a couple of weeks before her arrival, Dr Anderson, the Principal Medical Officer at Balaklava General hospital, gave evidence to Dr Andrew's Smith's First Commission, which had been initiated to examine the state of soldiers, hospitals and supplies. Smith had been so shocked and horrified at the reports coming back from the Crimea that in early November he sent the Deputy Inspector Alexander Cumming, his own assistant Dr Thomas Spence and Mr Maxwell, a barrister, to report. However, Dr Spence was unfortunately lost on the *Prince* during the Great Storm on 14 November and the Commission was delayed whilst awaiting his replacement, Staff Surgeon Patrick Laing. Dr Anderson complained of the hospital not being big enough for the number of patients he had (752 admitted in January 1855), where when the roof was not missing was in disrepair, there was no glass in the windows and 'The privies are abominable. It is unsuited for the treatment of sick. The smell of the drains is very offensive.'[112] Dr Anderson considered this effluence to be the cause of much fever and bowel complaints, which shows in official figures for that month. The Commissioners declared that Balaklava General hospital, formerly the village school, was capable of holding 101 patients, including extra marquees; we can already gain an idea of how overcrowded it must have been in the middle of the winter. Before the commissioners left, they noted how improvements were already being made and in February 1855, 421 soldiers were admitted; the highest number which then continued to steadily decrease until the end of the war. Of the 752 admitted in January, 239 were admitted for diarrhoea, 158 for continual fever, and 49 for cholera, which was closely followed by 45 for frostbite.[113]

Betsy describes nursing some of these frostbite injuries during her first few days at Balaklava General hospital, where she assisted in washing wounds and applying fresh poultices. The first wound she came across was to remove the bandages (which according to Betsy had not been changed from between two to six weeks) from a man's feet. All the toes fell off with the bandages. Another soldier had his hand fall off from the wrist. She also attended a shot wound with Dr Hanbury. The patient in question had been wounded at the Battle of Alma and a bullet had passed through him from front to back, narrowly missing his heart. The wound, which had not been dressed for five weeks, just below his shoulder blade contained 'a quart of maggots', which Betsy removed. She also noticed how well these men gradually recovered once their wounds were being attended to regularly. Betsy also remarked on the lack of beds, whereby most men were on trestles and boards with one blanket under them, one over and their great-coats, if they still had them, as pillows. There were no sheets. Besty then took it upon herself to go direct to the deputy-purveyor, Mr Fitzgerald, that evening to enquire after bedsteads and appropriate bedding. After he informed her that they had plenty, she requested they be put ready for the patients the next day, which they were. Besty then 'set the orderlies about washing, combing and changing the clothes of the poor men ...' and getting them into the beds. Although it seems highly unlikely Betsy did all this by herself, and that this could possibly be part of her autobiography that may be deemed dubious, it does correlate with the report from the First Commission, who stated that there were no sheets but '... the supply of bedsteads and bedding was sufficient'. Betsy goes onto say that she did indeed do it all be herself and '... the superintendent did not interfere. She just came and looked at what was going on. That was my Saturday's work, until twelve midnight.'[114]

By the beginning of October 1855, Betsy was joined at Balaklava General hospital by Bridgeman and all fifteen of her nuns. The Sisters of Mercy, with the blessing of their bishop, had made their decision to move from Koulali due to reduction in workload and the fact the hospital was about to be made over for the convalescing Sardinian troops.[11] Any serious nursing demand at Koulali had begun to deplete by August 1855; by this time, any ill and wounded soldiers were kept in the Crimean hospitals instead of being transferred to Scutari. Lord Raglan had ordered the extra Balaklava Castle hospital open for convalescents in April 1855, in addition to the General, where he had originally requested the eight nurses in January 1855, one being Betsy. Bridgeman felt they should be staying 'on mission' as she called it, and discussed with Miss Emily Hutton (Lady Superintendent at Koulali) about volunteering to go to the Crimea and the Balaklava General hospital. This came to nothing but after discussions with Father Woollett (who had replaced Father Ronan after he had returned home sick on 2 September 1855) acting as a go-between with the authorities, Dr John Hall was very much in favour of having the Sisters take charge of the nursing in Balaklava General hospital. The current Lady Superintendent, Miss Weare, would move to the Castle hospital for convalescents.[116]

Dr John Hall's dislike for FN in the Crimean War is well-known, although she returned the dislike in full force. John Hall FRS, MRCS, FRCS, M.D, KCB (1795 – 1866) had entered the Army Medical Service aged 20 in June 1815, after studying medicine at Guy's and St Thomas' hospitals in London. He was with the forces in Flanders against Napoleon and in 1817 left for Jamaica, where he spent the next nine years. He was promoted in 1822 to assistant-surgeon and by 1844 he had been promoted to Deputy Inspector-General of Hospitals and became a Fellow of the Royal College of Surgeons of England. In 1845, he earned his M.D at St Andrews University. Whilst deployed in Cape Town, South Africa in 1848, he met and married Lucy Campbell and she accompanied him to Bombay in 1851, where Hall initiated reforms in barrack accommodation and medical statistics. Throughout his medical career he was known as one of the most able officers known to colleagues; conscientious, not afraid of hard work and a man of action, not just words, as well as a stern disciplinarian but well respected by those in his charge.

He was still in Bombay when the War Office called him to the Crimea, arriving on 17 June 1854, his official title being Chief of the Medical Staff and, along with Dr Andrew Smith, became a scapegoat for all that went wrong in that first, dreadful winter of the Crimean War.[117] Hall had realised even before he arrived in the Crimea how unprepared Britain was for the war. His first task was to prepare Scutari barracks to become a hospital as well as looking at plans for extra beds, all with the disadvantage of arriving without time to make his own plans, policies or appointments, and having to accept what had already been put in place by Smith, from London and his medical officers such as Dumbreck who was in the Crimea. Smith had initially asked for a 5,000-bed capacity, an extra 20 per cent of the forces sent to war, in case of disease epidemics for example, which was ignored by the War Office. Smith did not relay this information to Hall as he knew he would realise 'it is an established thing [increasing bed capacity if needed], understood in the service …' and act accordingly.[118] Hall was only in Scutari for a week then went to Varna, Bulgaria where the fighting forces had been moved to, only to find a rising rate of death, disease and cholera. Sanitation in Varna was non-existent, bearing in mind this was the hot summer of 1854 and the general miasma theory of disease was prevalent. The toilets were trenches that were supposed to be 6-feet deep, covered by at least 6 inches of earth twice daily and used for only three days. None of this happened, leaving a mass of flies that landed on what food there was. Men washed in the rivers where they rinsed their clothes and where carcasses from the butchers were dumped; this was also the water used for cooking and drinking. Men that were ill, prostrate on the ground and dying of thirst, lapped from puddles left from animals. Medical treatments at the time included laxatives with mercury, the plant *ipecacuanha* as an emetic (no wonder dehydration was common), sinapisms (mustard plasters), fomentations (poultices) and enemas.[119]

The imperative supply chain to Scutari of bedding, iron beds, surgical supplies, medicines and stores was crippled by a number of factors. Although Hall had initiated 1,000 beds for Dr Menzies, the Principal Medical Officer, to work with, Smith had taken it upon himself to order the supplies for another 5,000. These supplies were diverted to Varna where they stayed, even after the army had moved on, due to the impassability of the environment, lack of a usable transport system and the need to look after the men that could still fight. There was then a huge fire in early August that decimated more supplies:

> '*10 August:* 10 p.m. A fire is raging in the town, and spreading rapidly. The commissariat stores evidently are on fire, which will baffle all previous arrangements, and we shall starve in the meantime ...
>
> *11 August:* Fire out this evening; our chief loss in biscuit, grain, and men's shoes. Five Greeks were caught setting fire to buildings by the French, who immediately bayoneted them. They do things better than we do in this way.[120]

Then you had the ill-equipped, under-staffed and not-fit-for-purpose Purveyor's department. As early as June, Dr Menzies had complained to Hall about the 68-year-old Mr Ward, head purveyor at Scutari, and his lack of accounts, refusing or ignoring requisitions and Dr Menzies recommended him being declared medically unfit and be invalided home. Ward, however, had friends in high places and after an appeal, Lord Raglan – without meeting or knowing Ward – overruled these concerns insisting he stay in post. It was the purveyor's department that became the bugbear of both FN and Betsy.[121]

Although letters between Hall and FN remained polite, even FN's first official biographer, Sir Edward Cook's sympathies appear to lie with Hall: 'To me, after much reading of the documents, it seems that Dr. Hall was the victim of a false position. He had been appointed Medical Inspector-General in the Crimea when he was still in India, and he did not arrive on the scene in time to think out the preparations properly.'[122] Twenty years earlier, Hall had been an advocate for female nurses in military hospitals, but considered the Crimean experiment extravagant. Sidney Herbert, writing to Dr Cumming (Deputy Inspector) in November 1854 also acknowledged that:

> The authorities of the hospital have been attacked without consideration for their difficulties, and have no doubt been inclined to refuse assistance, thinking its offer conveyed an imputation. The French, I am told, are wiser, and accept for their hospitals everything which is offered to them. The first object should be to make the hospital as good and the people in it as comfortable as it is possible to do.

Hall, however, had a reputation for not accepting help, especially after negative reports in the press and by philanthropic visitors to the area such as Reverand Osborne and Augustus Stafford. Herbert wrote to Lord Raglan in December 1854, stating that

> I cannot help feeling that Dr. Hall resents offers of assistance as being slurs on his preparations. The exaggerated attacks of *The Times* make him take refuge in secrecy, instead of meeting them by exertions to remedy deficiencies which must exist under the circumstances, and which are, therefore, no discredit if everything is done to repair them.[124]

Bridgeman and her nuns arrived at Balaklava General hospital on 12 October and was shown around the hospital the next day. She notes in her diary the seven wards in the stone building of the General hospital were comfortable, but the fourteen wards set up in the huts were awful. She then addresses the extra diet kitchen, Besty's domain, which Bridgeman describes as a 'most discreditable establishment' with 'filth and disorder at every side'. It is also at this part of Bridgeman's story where she gives us a description of the nurse in sole charge of the kitchen, a 'hard-working, honest old woman but quite a character, who did just what she pleased in it'.[124] Bridgeman then writes about the system of cooking and diet for the sick, calling Betsy 'Mrs Davis'. Betsy, who was becoming unwell at this point and had already decided to go home, notes in her autobiography that she cooked for the Sisters of Mercy on their arrival and also inspected some bales of shirts with Mrs Bridgeman and Sister Mary Chaucer that were being stored in the kitchen for want of storage space elsewhere. This shows that Betsy and Bridgeman certainly met, even though the pair did not work together for very long, as Betsy would go home at the beginning of November. In her book on the Sisters of Mercy, Bolster incorrectly notes that 'Mrs Davis never worked with the Sisters of Mercy in the Crimean military hospitals. She only knew of them by repute.'[125] And although Betsy and Bridgeman also travelled from London to the Crimea together, it is highly likely Bridgeman kept her nuns as far from the working-class nurses as possible.

# Chapter 7

# Going Home

## Betsy Cadwaladyr

Out of the three ladies discussed in this book, the first to leave the Crimea and return to England was Betsy. She had begun to feel unwell in October 1855, as she mentions while discussing the arrival of the Sisters of Mercy at Balaklava General hospital. She also states that she was suffering from diarrhoea and an attack of dysentery; one must remember her age and how hard she had worked. She was at least in her mid to late sixties at this point and exhaustion would have made her vulnerable to the many infections and diseases around her. FN did not want her to go, having seen how good she was at supplying the soldiers with a solid, healing diet (even being lavish with supplies and not caring one iota on what amount should – or should not – be allowed!).

FN went to visit Betsy on a couple of occasions at Balaklava, travelling on the same ship from Scutari and Koulali to join the Sisters of Mercy as they transferred to Balaklava in early October, when we know Betsy was unwell. According to Betsy's autobiography, she had several meetings with FN, who asked her about certain nurses' behaviour, rule-breaking – if any – and procedures at both Balaklava General and the other hospital that had been opened, Castle hospital, up the hill from the General. Betsy confirmed what nurses she knew, refused to speak about those she did not and asked

## Going Home

FN to leave her kitchens when she was busy. It was around this time Betsy announced to Dr John Hall that she wished to go home due to her health issues, although he wanted her to go somewhere warm and clean to recuperate such as Malta or South of France and advised FN Betsy was unwell. Betsy, however, not wanting to die in a foreign land, was adamant she was going home.

Although FN offered to send Betsy to the places recommended by Dr Hall at her own expense, Betsy refused and FN ended up paying Betsy minimal wages, although she did recommend Betsy have twelve months' wages when home. FN then offered to sort passage on the next ship home, which Betsy refused. Despite this, FN named a ship for her in a letter to Miss Weare, who went to approve the ship but seeing Betsy would be the only female aboard, Miss Weare refused her to sail. Betsy's dislike of FN is obvious, and it is doubtful anything FN did would have moved Betsy, the woman she had determined not to like before she even met her.[1]

As it turned out, Betsy spoke to the harbour master, whom she names as Captain Heath, herself, and secured a passage on the ship *Calcutta,* setting sail in early November 1855; there was indeed a Captain Heath, responsible for Balaklava harbour with two other Captains under Admiral Berkeley.[2] Betsy notes she sailed out of the Crimea on Saturday, 3 November 1855 and we do know the *Calcutta* arrived in Malta on 18 November on her way home to Portsmouth, docking there on 7 December to 'land her invalids'.[3] We know Betsy lived in poverty after returning from the Crimea and that FN's request for her wages were not honoured, nor were her letters of recommendations from Miss Weare (who had been Superintendent of Nurses at Balaklava and whom Betsy had been fond of), Dr Hadley, medical officer at Balaklava and the Purveyor in Chief, Mr David Fitzgerald. There was also the appeal for funds from her biographer, Jane Williams, at the end of the book: 'NOTICE. In the decline of life and broken health, the Heroine of this narrative is left unprovided for. She is anxious to obtain employment in some public institution, and is still fully capable of executing any office of trust and vigilant inspection ...'[4]

Betsy passed away on 17 July 1860 aged 72 from an abdominal abscess and, as we saw in an earlier chapter, was buried in a pauper's grave that has now been rectified and recognised. Although we know from the 1851 census and her own autobiography that Betsy was living with her sister in East Road, Shoreditch before she went to the Crimea, she died at her home at 22 Herbert Street, Hoxton (next to Shoreditch parish). This area was a poverty-stricken demographic by 1860 and was the fastest growing London suburb in the nineteenth century due to being a hub for furniture making, which led to the creation of a myriad of slum housing. Although it no longer exists, Herbert Street was not too far from where Betsy had lived with her sister Bridget before the Crimean War and would have been just slightly south of what it now Shoreditch Park. Herbert Street sat between Wenlock Street and Murray Street (now Murray Grove), which still exist albeit rebuilt; this area can be found on Charles Booth's interactive poverty maps for comparison.[5]

## Sister Mary Francis Bridgeman

The next to go home was Mother Bridgeman and her Sisters of Mercy. On 24 February 1856, the Paris Peace Conference finally happened and Armistice Day was declared five days later, on 29 February. This raised great hope within Bridgeman that the war would stop and she, along with her Sisters, could end their mission and return home. However, on 16 March, General Orders (published directives from the Commander to the soldiers under his command) were issued for a ceasefire in respect of the peace talks, included in which was a clarification of FN's role as Superintendent of Nursing and that FN was to be recognised as the 'General Superintendent of the female nursing establishment in the military hospitals of the army'. No nurse of any denomination was to be moved or introduced to the hospitals in the East without FN's clearance, although FN herself was ordered to have the approval of the principal medical officers of any decision regarding nursing and his orders would come through FN only.[6] As Bridgeman wrote in her diary, this system was liable to fail as it took at least a fortnight for any written correspondence to arrive from Scutari, where FN was based. However, this was not a major concern for her as by this time, with peace around the corner, Bridgeman had decided that if she could not work under Hall on the terms the Sisters had when they had first transferred to Balaklava at his request five months earlier, then she would go home and consider the Sisters of Mercy mission complete. Sister M. Croke wrote that FN turned up at the Balaklava General hospital on 25 March to announce the clarification of her role with the General Order; Sister M. Doyle wrote that as nearly all the patients were convalescents and peace was about to be announced, the Sisters of Mercy were happy to return home before the crush of the disbanding military, as well as patients and medical staff, all of whom would need to sail back to England. The Sisters of Mercy were completely loyal to their Mother Superior.[7]

FN wasted no time in seeking out Bridgeman, going to see her the day she arrived at the hospital and getting straight to the point; she wanted the Sisters to stay nursing at Balaklava General. FN was more than happy to trust the opinion of Dr Beatson, the medical officer, who had told her how much gratitude the doctors owed the Sisters, as well as the satisfaction of Dr Hall.[8] On the surface, this initial meeting looks like FN was making a concerted effort due to the strained relations between the two so far and indeed, she was polite, official and happy for them to continue their nursing. Despite everything, FN never had cause to complain about Bridgeman's standard of nursing and did not wish to change it, only to make alterations to the administration of the place. She did, however, write a letter about her mistrust of the Roman Catholics to Lieutenant Colonel Lefroy, an army officer and meteorologist who had been made Scientific Advisor to the army in 1854 and in October 1855 was sent to the Crimea to investigate the conditions of the hospitals and staff in the East.[9] Lefroy became acquainted with FN and they worked together on army health reforms thereafter. In a letter dated 16 March 1856, she wrote: 'I have always said that a R.C [Roman Catholic] can do everything which we cannot do, lie, steal, murder, slander, because we are afraid of the Roman Catholics. What an advantage it must be!' Despite getting on well with Mother M. Moore and the English Sisters of Mercy, she wrote about the 'Bridgemans' at Balaklava being the 'tools of an Irish faction' due to their distrust of the British government. Interestingly, FN goes onto write that 'Above all, I am afraid of their resigning & making martyrs of themselves, which is their grand object'. This says more about her polite request to Bridgeman than anything else, although FN was correct when she says that 'having none other than Roman Catholics nursing in one hospital goes against the War Office's initial instructions'. At that time, however, that initial directive did not include Balaklava.[10] The Irish Sisters of Mercy had no intention of making themselves martyrs; in fact, Bridgeman did not retaliate publicly against the complaints raised about the hospital at Balaklava in the Sanitary Commission of 1858, and none of the Sisters' diaries was published in full until after the death of the last surviving one, Sister M. Doyle, in 1908.

Bridgeman had not particularly helped herself; when a much-loved member of their group, Sister Winifred, died from cholera shortly after the Sisters' arrival at Balaklava, FN fetched a priest at Bridgeman's request and also stayed up all night with them to help guard Sister Winifred's body against rats as until a coffin was made, the burial could not commence. In the three extant diaries of the Sisters of Mercy, Sister Doyle only mentions FN attending the funeral and joining in the prayers, while Sister Croke notes that FN fetched the priest and joined in prayers, and Bridgeman states she joined in prayers and tried to help arrange the burial site but felt FN was performing surveillance. Maybe FN came over as controlling, but that was her personality and as Bridgeman was of a similar type, she would not see it as kindness. Much is written of Bridgeman's refusal to accept FN's offer of arranging a headstone. In fact, the 89th Regiment, an Irish regiment, had offered first and was gladly accepted by Bridgeman, so some interactions between the two need to be occasionally tempered with a further look at the bigger picture.[11]

On 28 March 1856, Bridgeman wrote to Hall that, 'As I find it is no longer in your power to keep us here on the terms on which you accepted our services in the Crimea, I beg to resign my charge to you from whom I received it.' Hall replied that, 'I cannot permit you, and the Sisters under your direction, to leave the Crimea, without an expression of the high opinion I entertain of your administration, and of the very important aid you have rendered to the sick under your care.' General Codrington, who had been commander in chief of the Crimean War since November 1855, wrote to Hall saying, 'I request you to assure that lady of the high estimation in which her services, and those of the Sisters, are held by us all; founded as that opinion is on the experience of yourself, the medical officers of the hospital, and of the many patients, both wounded and sick who ... have benefited by their care.'[12] Hall found Bridgeman and her Sisters transport home and on Friday, 11 April 1856, they boarded the *Cleopatra*, ready to sail at 4pm the next day. About an hour after boarding, FN arrived on deck to discuss a handover, admonishing Bridgeman for not updating details about their departure. Bridgeman declared she had notified Hall and was only answerable to him. FN then asked for the keys as the purveyor, Mr Fitzgerald – also no fan of FN and vice versa – informed FN he did not have them. Bridgeman replied she had put the keys in the hands of a reliable orderly named Brennan, who obviously had not finished dealing with the stores and thus had not handed them over to Fitzgerald just yet. It would have been very interesting to watch this exchange of these two highly intelligent, strong-witted but no doubt exhausted women.

The next day, Saturday, 12 April, the *Cleopatra* sailed from Balaklava bound for Portsmouth, where they would then board a train for a convent in London and then home to their various convents, Bridgeman's being Kinsale in Ireland. They finally docked in Portsmouth on Thursday, 8 May, an event detailed in Sister Croke's diary. Their homecoming is also detailed in Bolster's book *The Sisters of Mercy in the Crimean War*, where she goes onto say that the officer in charge of the regiment (the Army Works Corps) who had come home on the same ship, invited the Sisters to walk the short distance with them to the railway station, at the head of the regiment. This they did to the cheering crowds, although Bolster goes onto say, 'Their compliance with the officer's request shows how little the events of the Crimean War had helped to water down the anti-Catholic prejudices of England, for with woeful lack of chivalry and appreciation the crowd began to hoot and pelt the Sisters until the soldiers lifted their rifles to the rescue.'[13] She references this statement to one of the three surviving Sisters of Mercy diaries, written by Sister M Croke. However, Croke only describes the arrival home and the journey to London, with no mention given of being harassed by the crowds. Indeed, none of the contemporaneous diaries mentions this situation. Newspapers reporting the arrival of the *Cleopatra* confirm 511 men of the Army Works Corp, two surgeons and eleven Sisters of Mercy arrived in Portsmouth on that day but again, there is no mention of any harassment.[14] Once docked, the Sisters of Mercy caught the train to London, arriving at 9pm at the Sisters of Mercy Convent in Blandford Square (near Marylebone) at about 10pm.

Within a week of the departure of the Sisters of Mercy, on 17 April FN wrote home to her Uncle Sam, who was helping her with her finances. In the letter she declared:

Your pigsty is cleaner than our Quarters or than the wards of the Hospital, as left by Mrs Bridgeman. The patients were grimed with dirt, infested with vermin with bedsores like Lazarus,

## Going Home

(Mrs Bridgeman, I suppose, thought it holy) ... Dr John Hall visited the Hospital and wrote an angry letter, saying that he was 'disgusted with the state of the Hospital' & 'ordered it all to be put back into the admirable order it was in previously'.[15]

By now, FN was very tired by the situation and it must be considered that these statements were exaggerated as explanations given for these accusations are noted in correspondence from Bridgeman to Dr Hall. The fact remains that the death rate in Balaklava General hospital dropped from October 1855 to the end of the conflict (June 1856) to just 2 per cent. Out of those nine months, seven were under the nursing direction of the Sisters of Mercy alone.[16] Bridgeman would later write to Dr John Hall privately in 1858 reputing these claims that were showcased in the Sanitary Commission, giving explanations for each accusation, explanations which were also confirmed and supported by medical staff. In the government's Sanitary Commission of 1858, FN declared Balaklava hospital a disaster from the day she entered it and Bridgeman's Sisters of Mercy had left, on 11 April 1855. She declared that the orderlies were drunk, extra bedding and clothing cluttered up the wards and a patient, suffering from frostbite and bed sores, was left neglected for weeks with undiscovered wounds on his back.[17] The exacting letter Bridgeman wrote to Hall was to be used only if needed and was never published. She explained that under FN's own direction dating from January 1855 at Scutari, no wounds were to be dressed by female nurses, only by the medical dressers. Bridgeman also goes onto say that they acted only under the guidance of the medical officers and she knew the patient's wounds were dressed regularly as the Sisters prepared the linen for said wounds: 'The dressings, usually five in number – two for the back, two for the feet and one for the hip – she [the Sister assisting the doctor] saw these going on and heard the piteous complaints of the sufferer.'[18] This also shows the Sisters were aware of every wound on the patient and were acting under doctor's instructions only, as they were instructed to do.

In 1856, on her return from the Crimea, Bridgeman was made Mistress of Novices at her convent in Kinsale and on the departure of the current Mother Superior to America in 1858, Bridgeman was elected Mother Superior of Kinsale and was to be re-elected every six years until her death in 1888. She worked closely with children in poverty until she became unwell with what was likely a form of cancer, as described by Bolster in *Sisters of Mercy:* 'A malignant growth began slowly but surely to gnaw its insidious way through her system ...weeks and months of excruciating agony saw her practising those virtues of patience and resignation ... she had encouraged in others ... The end came peacefully on February 11, 1888 ...'[19]

## Florence Nightingale

FN stayed in Balaklava until the end of June 1856, with her last letter from there dated the 27th. She had been feeling exhausted again and, convinced she was going to die, wrote to General Storks on 10 May to ask him to carry out her last requests, supporting her in death as he had in life.[20] A letter presumed to have been written home to the Bracebridges on 30 May 1856 states that some of the nurses and all the unwell soldiers had been sent home first, while a letter to her sister dated 2 June notes that '... all her invalided sons' had gone home. FN was to stay until her last nurse had departed with the remaining 41,000 troops awaiting the men-at-war ships from England to carry them back. FN declined the offer of transport home aboard a warship, instead wanting and needing to travel incognito under the alias of Miss Smith, with her Aunt Mai aboard the *Danube,* sailing from Constantinople around 28 July 1856. She had written to her family on 17 July to update them about arrangements to come home, but stayed deliberately vague exactly when that would be so her family, when pestered by the papers or the public, could say with all honesty they did not know when she was returning.

Possibly her final letter from the East was to her good friend Sister Gonzaga from the Bermondsey Sisters of Mercy, dated 23 July, advising of some last accounts and that she would keep her promise to call in to the convent when she arrived back; this would be a much welcome visit for pleasure, not business, and FN planned to sneak away quietly from Bermondsey to return home to Lea Hurst in Derbyshire. She did indeed keep her promise; after a stopover in Paris on 4 August, she arrived in England on the 7th, visiting the Sisters for a few hours before embarking on a train home to Derbyshire, with Aunt Mai departing to Surrey. FN quite literally walked in on her family home unannounced, much to the surprise of her immediate family. Her sister Parthe made sure she got the rest and peace she so desperately needed after nearly two years away from home in a war zone, spending many of those months dealing with miscommunications, out of date and faulty arrangements, the tragic death after death of the soldiers and handling those who had taken offence at her mission, her person and her authority. Rest was needed and 'seclusion to hide herself from publicity and applause. The world praised her self-sacrifice. She felt she had made none.'[21]

FN had indeed made sacrifices, but not in the way she may have realised at the time. Her own health issues would have knock-on effects for her until at least 1888. Whilst visiting the Balaklava hospitals in early May 1855, and shortly after visiting Betsy in her kitchen with the chef Soyer, FN suddenly fell ill whilst on board her ship. She had arrived on 5 May and on her thirty-fifth birthday, 12 May, was hit by a sudden fever and fatigue to the point where she was unable to walk. This date, strangely not mentioned by her original biographer Cook, can be corroborated by Betsy's mention of the visit by FN and Soyer to her Balaklava kitchen. FN landed in the Crimea on 5 May 1855 (a Saturday) and Betsy says she did not meet her until the Friday after her arrival, which would have been 11 May. Betsy mentions that the next day, FN had a violent quarrel with the nurse Mrs Disney, who was drunk, and on that same day, FN was taken ill on board her ship and transported by guardsmen in a litter, as a patient, to Balaklava Castle hospital. FN was considered to be at death's door with Crimean Fever until 22/24 May when she returned to Scutari, weak and pale.

During the time she was laid low, FN could not eat, suffered a recurring fever that led to delirium and spoke in nothing but a whisper for a couple of weeks.[22] Five months later, she returned to the Crimea; this would have been early October as we have seen she travelled with the Sisters of Mercy when they left Koulali to nurse independently under Hall. Whilst there, FN had an attack of sciatica and was resting in hospital for week, returning to Scutari at the end of November, still suffering symptoms from her fever such as earache and insomnia.[23] There is a description of FN from a gathering at the Ambassador's house in Therapia on Christmas Day 1855, where FN attended and a fellow guest wrote of her:

> She is very slight, rather above the middle height; her face is long and thin, but this may be from recent illness and great fatigue. She has a very prominent nose, slightly Roman; and small dark eyes, kind, yet penetrating; but her face does not give you at all the idea of great talent. She looks a quiet, persevering, orderly, lady-like woman. She was still very weak, and could not join in the games ...[24]

A couple of weeks before that Christmas, Sister Terrot, one of the Devonport Sellonite Sisters, and an admirer of FN, wrote

> On returning to our quarters, we found ourselves shut out, as the nurses had retired to rest. However, on our ringing, Miss Nightingale herself opened the door, and on hearing our story, she searched out some provisions and sent us back with them to our poor exhausted friend, and remained up to let us in on our return. She looked, I thought, very sweet and kind, though delicate and worn out.[25]

According to some sources, her ongoing symptomatic illness caused FN to become obsessed at failing in her mission in the Crimea, which would explain her pedantic and frustrated behaviour with Hall and Fitzgerald after the departure of the Sisters of Mercy, which lasted more or less until Balaklava ceased being a military hospital at the end of June 1856 (although even Bridgeman had initial struggles with Fitzgerald). In fact, Sidney Herbert was prompted to write to her on 6 March 1856 to urge her to relax:

> And now I am going to scold you. You have been done with your long, anxious, harassing work. You see jealousness and meanness all around you. You hear of one-sided, unfair, and unjust reports made of your proceedings, and of those under you. But you overrate their importance, you attribute too much motive to them, and you write upon them with an irritation and a vehemence detracts very much from the weight which would otherwise attach to what you say.[26]

FN replied on 3 April, reminding him that while he wrote from Belgrave Square, she was writing from a Crimean hut and had received his letter late one cold, frosty night after being on foot and horseback for fifteen hours, mostly with no food.[27] At this point, FN was suffering insomnia, nausea and chronic fatigue that would haunt her for over thirty years.

It is well known how hard FN worked on nursing and sanitary reform when back from the Crimea, firstly on military health and hospitals and then with a passion for sanitary conditions, in public health as much as anywhere else. She never actually performed hands-on nursing again but was a prolific writer and advisor with everyone seeking her opinion on health matters as well as her work as a statistician. In August and September 1857, FN had her first chronic illness relapse, with fever, palpitations, tachycardia, depression and joint pains and by the end of 1857, both FN and her family thought it highly probable she would die.[28] She was inspired to work harder by thinking she had less time to do it in, which would account for her phenomenal output of work over the years she was a self-secluded invalid.

It has been suggested this workload undertaken whilst FN was unwell could be a sign of bipolar disorder and although we have seen she was prone to depression before going to the Crimea, her symptoms are much more aligned with severe, recurrent attacks of Brucellois caused by the bacteria *Brucella melitensis,* firstly identified in 1887, although symptoms had been accurately described back in 1861 by an Army medical doctor, including tachycardia and restlessness with some form of rheumatism that would recur as further chronic attacks.[29] If depression was also a symptom and FN had bouts of depression before the Crimea, it is highly possible, and understandable, that mixed into the organic nature of her post-Crimea illness, there were also mental health issues to contend with. Studies have shown that FN possibly had PTSD; thirty years of chronic attacks of headaches, depression and invalidism are protracted even for *Brucella melitensis*, and these symptoms appeared to have stopped from 1888 onwards.[30] However, in 1887, she considered herself 'almost blind' and it was known her memory was failing by 1895. From this time, she hardly left her house on South Street, Mayfair due to her frailty and lost her ability to write almost instantly, although she still enjoyed occasional visits by nurses from St Thomas' Hospital. From 1901 she could neither read nor write at all anymore and by the autumn of 1909, FN was struggling to 'give attention to anything without great effort'. From February 1910, she was completely blind and her understanding of anything was 'feeble'.

FN fell asleep around noon on 13 August 1910 and died in her sleep around 2.30pm, surrounded by a couple of family members and her nurse. Interestingly, her death certificate was signed by Dr Louisa Garrett Anderson M.D, daughter of Dr Elizabeth Garrett Anderson, the first woman to qualify as a physician and surgeon in Britain in 1865. The cause of death was given as old age and heart failure, but aged 90 years and three months, FN had outlived all her immediate family.[31]

One can only imagine the horrors and situations these three remarkable, self-sacrificing women saw during not only the Crimean War, but in their lifetimes. All lived to a good age considering what they dealt with for years, although the health conditions shown above such as frailty and some form of dementia are just as common today. The poverty, lack of sanitation and the lack of understanding of hygiene these ladies lived through is beyond the scope of our modern minds. And yet, in the grand scheme of things, we are not looking back too far in time when these horrors abounded. A nursing career without safe pain relief, antibiotics and routine hygienic practice is a phenomenon that will continue to fascinate and demand to be studied and written about.

# Appendix 1

# ADAPTED FROM MASLOW'S HEIRARCHY OF NEEDS

| | |
|---|---|
| **PHYSIOLOGICAL DRIVES**<br><br>**When these drives are satisfied, higher needs emerge**<br>↓ | HUNGER<br>THIRST<br>SEX |
| **SAFETY NEEDS** | Being healthy, safe childhood & protected from danger & violence, financially stable, familiarity. |
| **LOVE NEEDS** | Giving & receiving love & affection, belonging, affectionate relationships with people in groups, family units & people in general. |
| **ESTEEM NEEDS** | Self-confidence, strength, capability, being useful & necessary. |
| **SELF-ACTUALISATION** | Individualised & subjective, a desire for self-fulfilment & to realise one's full potential such as creativity. |

# Appendix 2

# Scutari & Koulali Hospitals
# January 1855

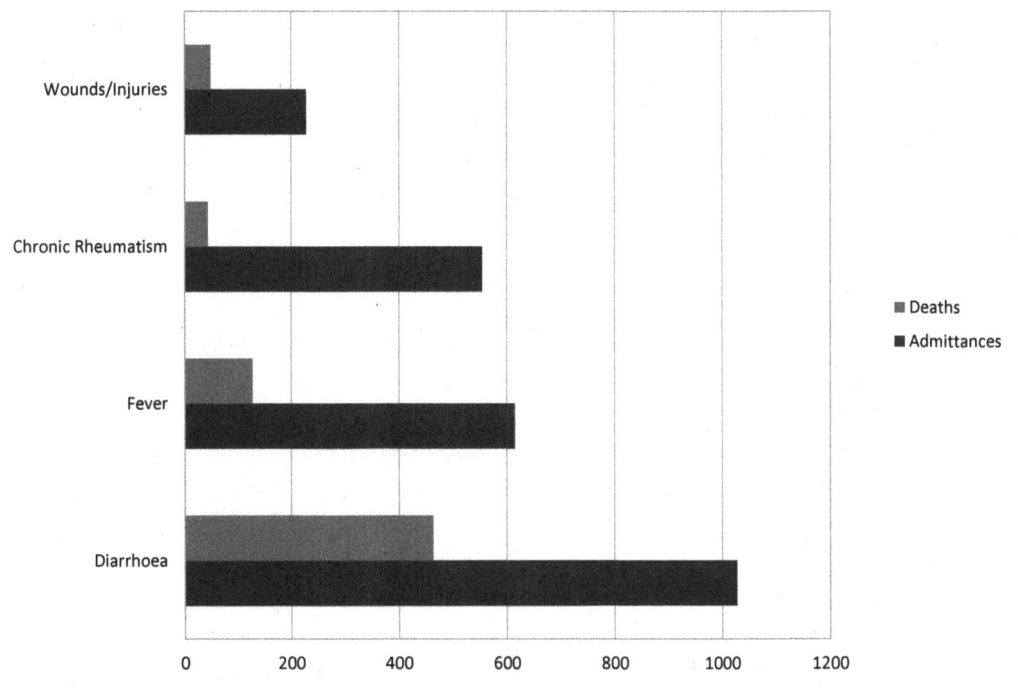

# NOTES

## Introduction

1. Meehan (2003) p.100
2. Wyatt (2019) p.10; Kleisiaris *et al*
3. Clarridge, p.187; Powell [essay]; Clark [blog article, 2014]
4. Sullivan, p.298
5. Luddy/Bridgeman, p.230
6. Notes on Nursing, p.9
7. Notes on Hospitals, p.49
8. Dock v3, p.86
9. Meehan (2012), p.2906; McDonald (2014), p.2426
10. Dock & Stewart (1920), p.260; p.373-8
11. McDonald (2014), p.2432

## Chapter 1: Nursing from Antiquity to Victorian England

1. Smith (1864), v3, pp.1016-17
2. Donohue, p.72
3. Kleisiaris *et al*
4. Jones, pp.124-5; Frank, p.45; Donohue, pp.72-4
5. Rosedahl & Kowalski, pp.1-2; Wyatt, pp.7-9
6. Bostock & Riley, v5, p.357; Sabatini p.391

## Notes

7. Nutting & Dock, v1, p.30
8. Charaka-Samhita, chapter 9 (online)
9. Nutting & Dock, v1, pp.32-3; Charaka-Samhita, Chapter 15 (online)
10. Minkowski, p.289
11. Sabatini, p.393; Power (1926), p.422
12. Dock & Stewart, p.xviii; Frank, pp.79-80; Donahue, pp.125-8
13. Frank p.84-5
14. Huggon, p.35
15. Jameson (1890), pp.58-9
16. Historic England; Atkinson - The Cartulary of Whitby pp.517-19; Clay, p.75
17. Carlin pp.22-4; Rubin, pp.41-57
18. Page (1906) at British History Online
19. CPR 1281-1292, p.113
20. CPR 1281-1292, p.114; Also see CClR 1272-1279, p.86 & Page *ibid.*
21. Knowles, 1963, p.484
22. Gaweda, pp.31-5; For articles on the Church Councils, see *Papal Encyclicals Online*
23. Mount, 2016, pp.34-7
24. Page (1974) at British History Online.
25. CPR 1334-1338, pp.266-8; Carpenter (2015) ed. Cartulary of St Leonard's Hospital, pp.xli – xlii
26. Cullum, pp.13-15; Rawcliffe (1996), pp.113-14; Stell, p.5
27. Dock & Stewart (1920) p.376
28. ODNB; Bucknill, pp.174-5; Wyatt p.30; Doubleday & Page (1903) at British History Online.
29. Wilkinson, p.lxiii, pp.xcvii-iii; Walcott, M (1868) pp.272-3; CPR 1221, pp.322-3
30. Giles, (1847), p.453; Hilton, p.47-8
31. Rawcliffe (2002), p.158
32. Wyatt, p.36; www.rfsk.org.uk/history; Rawcliffe (2002), p.159; Donohue, p.175
33. Jessopp & James (1896), p.31; Rawcliffe (1995), pp.41-2, p.45

34. The Home-life of English Ladies in the XVII Century, p.163
35. *Ibid*, p.167; Fitzalan-Howard, pp.311-12; Nutting & Dock et al, v1, p.467
36. Bolton, p.333
37. Rawcliffe (1997), p.206; Rawcliffe (1995), p.113
38. Minkowski, p.289; https://www.florence-nightingale.co.uk/florence-in-her-own-words-germ-theory/
39. Murphy-Hiscock, pp.18-19
40. World Health Organisation (2019)
41. Carmoner & Pereira pp.379-85
42. Gaweda, p.61-2; Jonsen, p.13-16; Rubin, p.41-57
43. Frank, p.88; Walsh (1911), pp.150-1 - *see also* chapter 6
44. Green (2006), p.50
45. Power (1975) pp.78-80; Green (2006), pp.49-62
46. Conrad *et al*, p.236, p.463
47. Hunter (1834), pp.7-43
48. Donahue, p.188
49. Frank, p.126
50. Wyatt, p.39; Donahue, pp.188-90
51. Thomas More (1516), p.59
52. Wyatt, p.23; Frank, p.68-9; Nutting & Dock, v1, p.124
53. Wyatt, p.39
54. Clarke (2016)
55. Donahue, p.193
56. Wyatt pp.43-45; Nutting & Dock, v1, *see* chapter 14
57. Nolan (1786), pp.11-13
58. Nutting & Dock, v1, p.p510-12
59. Nutting & Dock, v1, p.536
60. Dickens (2010), p.xxix
61. Dickens (2010), p.313
62. Summers (1989), p.372
63. ODNB
64. ODNB; Barnard, pp.12-14
65. White (1978), pp.20-1; p.30

*Notes*

66. Twining (1898), p.85
67. Twining (1898), p.82, pp.76-7
68. Twining (1898), p.29
69. Twining (1866), p.15
70. Nurses and Doctors (1880). Anon
71. Redpath

## Chapter 2: Crimean Call to Nurses

1. Cook, v1, p.148
2. Aloysius, Sister (1897) Memories of the Crimea by Sister Mary Aloysius
3. Hodkinson (2022); Helmstadter (2020), p.31; Page (1909), pp.546-9; Hinton (2019), p.75
4. Cantlie, v1, p.26, p.500
5. Manuscripts of Duke of Portland, p.309
6. CSP Dom (1653), no.81, p.177; Manwaring, p.82
7. Shepherd, v1, p.15
8. CSP Dom (1652-3), p.484, p.490
9. CSP Dom (1654), p.447, p.456
10. CSP Dom (1655), p.159
11. Manwaring, p.90
12. MacDonald (1935), p.119
13. National Army Museum at www.nam.ac.uk/crimea; Fisher (2004)
14. Woodham-Smith, p.82
15. Dr Andrew Smith (1858), Preface in *Medical & Surgical History Volume 1*
16. Goldie, p.16
17. Bolster, p.2
18. Helmstadter (2020), p.34
19. Goldie, p.16
20. Windham (1897), p.17
21. Hansard (12/12/1854), Colonel Dunne, Volume 136, Column 195-7

22. Dr Andrew Smith (1858), pp.40-3 in *Medical & Surgical History Volume 1*
23. Usherwood Journal, Part 4
24. Reid (1911), p.9
25. Russell (1858), pp.3-4
26. Cook, v1, p.146
27. Shepherd, v2, p.419
28. Cantlie, v1, p.45
29. Helmstadter (2020), p.18
30. Lawson (1858), p.8
31. Figes, pp.216-18; Russell (1858), p.63
32. Goldie, p.17
33. Helmstadter (2020), p.19
34. Windham (1897), p.29
35. Helmstadter (2020), p.18
36. Cook, v1, p.149
37. Helmstadter (2020) *see* Chapter 7; Farmer, pp.292-3; Jameson (1857), pp.47, 59-60; www.filles-de-la-charite.org
38. Aloysius, p.31
39. Hendricks *et al* (2014), pp.222-4; Figes, p.296
40. Figes, pp.298-9
41. Shepherd, v1, p.215; Connor, pp.192-3; *Medical & Surgical History Volume II*, pp.368-9; Maxwell (1855), p.197
42. White (2014), p.114; Edwards (2013), p.4
43. Skandalakis *et al*, p.1396; Sams (2015) at www.rcseng.ac.uk; White (2014), p.114
44. Sorokina, pp.59-60
45. Hendricks *et al* (2021) pp.9-18
46. Duke of Newcastle Speech 1854 in *Jameson* (1857), pp.112-13
47. Shepherd, v2, p.473
48. Helmstadter & Godden (2011), p.xx
49. Roxburgh, pp.71-2; Brown (2018) article at www.historyroom.org
50. Roxburgh, p.80
51. Rappaport (2007), p.169; Brown *ibid*

52. Register of Nurses; Helmstadter & Godden, pp.91-3
53. Aloysius (1897); Luddy/Doyle, pp.27-8
54. DIB; Bolster, p.xvii
55. DIB; *sistersofmercy.ie*
56. Bolster, p.14; Carroll (1881), v2, pp.128-31
57. Luddy, p.247; Bolster, pp.38-9
58. Helmstadter (2020), p.138
59. Williams (1947), p.353
60. Helmstadter (2020), pp.48-9; ODNB; LMA H01/ST/SJ; Williams (1947), pp.350-1
61. Goldie, p.37
62. Brayshay & Pointon (1983); Gregory (2020)
63. Churchman's Companion, August 1849, pp.108-10
64. Kinglake, v7, p.147
65. Lindgrén & Neumann pp.1575-77
66. Hamley (1891), pp.165-8
67. Kinglake, v7, pp.142-7
68. Shepherd, v1, pp.246-7
69. Mitra, p.331
70. Terrot, p.37
71. Bell (1867), v2, p.224
72. Kinglake, v7, p.170; Shepherd, v1, pp.298-9
73. Lindgrén & Neumann pp.1579-80; Shepherd v1 p.247; Figes, pp.279-80; www.historic-shipping.co.uk

## Chapter 3: Mother M. Francis Bridgeman – short biography to 1854

1. Taylor (1857), p.153
2. DIB; *www.clarelibrary.ie/eolas/coclare/people/joanna_bridgeman.htm*
3. DIB; Irish Monthly Journal (1892)
4. Irish Monthly Journal, p.227

5. Bolster, *see* Chapter 4
6. Irish Monthly Journal *ibid*
7. Aloysius, p.7
8. Bolster, pp.43-4
9. *Ibid*, p.45
10. Twining (1898), p.60
11. Rogers (1889), p.221
12. National Archives Ireland (2015) Survey of Hospital Archives in Ireland - hospital book v7; DIB; www.clarelibrary.ie

## Chapter 4: Betsy Cadwaladyr – short biography to 1854

1. Gwyneth Tyson Roberts, Dictionary of Welsh Biography.
2. ODNB; Yr Haul (May 1878), p.198; Saunderson (1836), p.15
3. Jones (2019), p.30
4. Helms (2020), p.62; Roberts (2019)
5. Jones (2019), p.40; LMA f60/1.1-f60/1.2 *see more at* https://cwfn.uoguelph.ca/archival/
6. Thorp (2015); AB, I, pp.50-8
7. *Ibid*, p.47
8. *Ibid*, pp.59-61; *see* Chapters 2-4
9. *Ibid*, p.84
10. Lloyds List (May 24, 1814), p.391; *see also* www.maritimearchives.co.uk
11. *The Cambrian* newspaper, 28 May 1814. Available at NLW, *see* https://newspapers.library.wales/view/3323265/3323268/12/perseverance
12. AB, I, p.77; Jones (2019), pp.13-15
13. AB, II, p.229
14. *Yr Haul,* May 1878, no.247 at NLW; burial records at http://www.goytrelocalhistory.org.uk/burials-chapel-ed-1882-1945/
15. *Yr Haul*, pp.196-8

16. AB, II, p239; *The Blue Books of 1847* (NLW); Reports of the Commissioners of Inquiry into the State of Education in Wales (1848), pp.403-404, p.536
17. *Ibid*, pp.239-40; Thorp (2015)
18. Helmstadter & Godden (2011), p.88; AB, II, pp.262-3
19. AB, II, p.239

## Chapter 5: Florence Nightingale – short biography to 1854

1. Goldie, p.184
2. White (2009)
3. *Ibid*; ODNB; History of Lea Hurst 2020 [article]; A Derbyshire Family [article]; Nightingale Family History [article]
4. Bostridge, p.23
5. *Ibid*, pp.38-9
6. Cook, v1, pp.14-15
7. O'Malley, p.112
8. Cook, v1, pp.44-5
9. O'Malley, p.113
10. ODNB; Riepel, pp.115-16; Bostridge, p.120; Cook, v1, pp.82-3
11. Donahue, pp.234-5; Waters, p.83; Nutting &Dock, v2, pp.1-4, p.33
12. Cook, v1, pp.92-3
13. Nightingale (1851), pp.16-17
14. Bostridge, p.154
15. ODNB; Bostridge, pp.183-4, p.186; O'Malley, chapter 10; Cook, v1, p.127
16. ODNB; Helmstadter (2020), pp.47-8; Huntsman *et al*, pp.350-80; The Nursing Record (1897) p.493; The British Medical Journal (1897) pp.1644-5; *The Institution for Nursing Sisters*, p.4, p.13
17. ODNB; Kyle, pp.13-15

18. Helmstadter & Godden (2011), p.77
19. *Ibid*, pp.75-84; Lost Hospitals of London; Lysons (1795)
20. Verney, pp.1-7
21. *Ibid*, pp.16-19; Helmstadter & Godden (2011), p.82
22. Verney, p.35
23. Helmstadter & Godden (2011), p.82
24. Lost Hospitals of London
25. Bostridge, p199, p.204-205
26. O'Malley, p216, p.224
27. Shepherd, pp.256-7; Bolster pp.14-16; Cook, v1, p.148-50; *see* www.peerage.com
28. Cook, v1, pp.150-1
29. *Ibid,* pp.152-3
30. Bostridge, p.209

## Chapter 6: Relationships in the Crimea

1. Stafford (*Hansard*, 29/1/1855, v136, column 1131-2)
2. Duke of Newcastle Speech, December 1854, (*Hansard*, v136, column 57)
3. Helmstadter (2020), p.42
4. Swift (1987) p.264, pp.273-4; Ralls (1974), pp.243-4
5. Bolster, pp.13-14
6. *Ibid*, p.180
7. Herbert (*Hansard*, 3/3/1854, v131, column 325)
8. Hagerty (2004), pp.23-4
9. Bolster, p.38
10. Herbert (*Hansard*, 15/12/1854, v136, column 376-8)
11. Luddy/Doyle, p.29
12. Cook, v1, p.249
13. Goldie, p.90
14. Luddy/Bridgeman, pp.150-1
15. Bolster, p.186-7

*Notes*

16. Goldie p.64 n13; p.144; Bolster, p.188
17. Goldie, p.155
18. Hagerty, p.30
19. Marrison (2022); Haralambos & Holborn, p.23; Cody (2021); Briggs, pp.276-7
20. Abel-Smith, p.5
21. Williams (2008), p.1462
22. Colonel Dunne (*Hansard*, 12/12/1854, v136, column 196)
23. ODNB; Collins (2016); Tyler (2001); Cook, v1, pp.148-9
24. ODNB; Shepherd, v1, p.36-44; *Hansard* (29/1/1855, v136, column 1135-9)
25. Cantlie, v2, p1
26. Goldie, p.62; O'Malley, p.267
27. Shep, v1, pp.38-9; O'Malley, p.267
28. ODNB; Hinton (2019), p.60; Shepherd, v1, pp.37-8; AMJ (May1855) pp.494-5
29. Helmstadter (2020), p5.3; Hinton (2019), p.60; Shepherd, v1 pp.37-8, p.79; Cantlie, v2, p12
30. Shepherd, v1, p.7; Millingen, p.14
31. Shepherd, v1, pp.5-6; Crumplin (2018)
32. Duke of Newcastle (*Hansard*, 12/12/1854, v136, c57
33. Goldie, pp.71-6
34. Luddy/Bridgeman, p.145; Luddy/Doyle, p.20; AB, p.266; Terrot, pp.37-8
35. Hinton (2019), p.61; Goldie, p.117
36. Helmstadter (2020) p.53-5; Shepherd, v1, p.37; Cook, v1, pp.224-5
37. Cantlie, v2, p.18; Sanitary Condition of the Army (1858), v2, Letters 6, 7 and 9, pp.2-3
38. Millingen, p.100
39. *Ibid*, p.112
40. *Ibid*, p.109
41. Cantlie, v1, pp.499-501
42. Helmstadter (2020), pp.49-50; Bostridge, p.217; Cook, v1, pp.158-60

43. Bostridge, pp.108-10
44. Canning Letters 8/2/1855 (private collection), *in* Shepherd, v1, p.271
45. Taylor (1857), p.7
46. Bostridge, p.236
47. *Ibid*; Helmstadter (2020), p.85
48. Luddy/Bridgeman, pp.123-4
49. Shepherd, v1, p.261; Bolster, p.27
50. Bolster, pp.27-8
51. Luddy/Doyle, p.6; Luddy, p.3
52. Luddy/Doyle, p.9; Bolster pp.31-2
53. Luddy/Bridgeman, p.123
54. *Ibid*, p.124; Bolster, p.59, p.115, p.178
55. Luddy/Bridgeman, p.122; Bolster, p.38
56. Luddy/Bridgeman, p.124
57. AB, II, p.241
58. Register of Nurses, p.14
59. AB *ibid*
60. Thorp (2015); Register of Nurses, *ibid;* AB, II, p.242
61. Taylor, pp.11-13
62. AB, II, pp.244-5
63. Luddy/Bridgeman, p.125
64. *Ibid,* pp.125-6; Taylor pp.13-17
65. Luddy/Doyle, p1.4
66. Taylor, pp.15-16
67. AB, II, p.245; Luddy/Doyle, p.14
68. Helmstadter (2020), p.211
69. AB, II, pp.247-8
70. Luddy, p.16; Lane-Poole, p.384; Bolster, p.75
71. Helmstadter (2020), p.116; Goldie, p.57; Cantlie, v2, p.127
72. Figes, p.55; Taylor, p.21
73. Luddy/Bridgeman, p.126
74. Luddy/Doyle, pp.16-17
75. Helmstadter (2020), p.203
76. Shepherd, v1, p.49

77. Penney, p.413
78. *Ibid*, p.417; Shepherd, v2, p.552
79. AB, II, p.252
80. Taylor, pp.26-7; AB, II, pp.250-2
81. AB, II, pp.251-3
82. Taylor, p.31-2
83. Luddy/Doyle, p.18
84. Goldie, pp.75, 78-9
85. Terrot, p.29
86. Shepherd, v1, p.316
87. Burfield, pp.56-7
88. Medical & Surgical History, v2, p.37
89. Shepherd, v2, pp.363-4; Taylor, pp.41-2
90. Cowen, p.4, pp.258-9
91. Taylor, p.200
92. Soyer (1857), pp.125-6
93. *Ibid*, p.524-5
94. *Ibid*, p.587-8
95. Nightingale (1858), Notes on matters affecting health ... p.408
96. Soyer, pp.162-3
97. AB, II, p281-2; Shepherd, v2, p.499
98. Goldie, p.6; Cantlie, v2, p.129; Terrot, p.101
99. Luddy/Doyle, p.18, pp.135-7; Doona, p.15; Carroll (1881), v2, p.132
100. Luddy/Bridgeman, p.138
101. AB, II, pp.252-3
102. *Ibid*, p.256; Taylor, p.36
103. Luddy/Bridgeman, p.205; Helmstadter & Godden (2011), pp.86-7; AB, II, p.294; Goldie, p.134; Register of Nurses, pp.14-16
104. Luddy/Bridgeman, pp.139-140; Bolster, pp.115-16
105. Bolster, pp.114-16; Goldie, p.80; Doona, p.15
106. Luddy/Bridgeman, pp.141-3; Taylor, pp.59-61

107. Shepherd, v2, p.578; Colborne & Brine, p.38, p.64; *Medical &Surgical History,* v1, p.518 and v2, p.253
108. *Medical & Surgical History,* v2, after p.481; See Appendix 2.
109. Shepherd, v2, pp.341-3, Cantlie, v2, p.128; Medical and Surgical History, v2, p.481
110. Taylor, p.39-40
111. Terrot, p.72
112. *First Commission* (1855), p.336; *Medical &Surgical History,* v2, p.483
113. Shep, v2, pp.374-5; *Medical & Surgical History,* v2, p.483; First Commission (1855) p.14-16
114. AB, II, pp.262-4; *First Commission* (1855), p.15
115. Luddy/Doyle, p.30; Luddy/Croke, p.75
116. Luddy/Bridgeman, pp.179-181; Goldie, p.156
117. ODNB; Shepherd, v1, pp.66-8; Cantlie, v2, p2.3
118. Cantlie, v1, p.24
119. *Ibid*, v2 pp.26-31
120. Bloy (2002)
121. Shepherd, v1, pp.168-170; Cantlie, v2, p.31-3
122. Cook, v1, p.288
123. Bostridge, p.287; Stanmore, v1, p.356, p.369
124. Luddy/Bridgeman, p.196
125. Bolster, p.175; AB, II, p.299

## Chapter 7: Going Home

1. AB, II, pp.298-300; Register of Nurses, p.14
2. *Hansard* (5/2/1855), v136, column 1271-2
3. AB, II, pp.300-1; Thorp (2015); *historic-shipping.co.uk*
4. AB, II, p.304, p.307-309
5. Thorp (2015); ODNB
6. Luddy/Bridgeman, p.222
7. Luddy/Doyle, p.47; Luddy/Croke, pp.101-102

*Notes*

8. Luddy/Bridgeman, p.223
9. Cook, v1, p.293; ODNB
10. Goldie, pp.230-1
11. Tastard, pp.95-6; Luddy/Doyle, pp.33-4; Luddy/Croke p.83; Luddy/Bridgeman, pp.197-8
12. Luddy/Doyle, pp.48-9; Luddy/Bridgeman, p.227
13. Bolster, p.272
14. Luddy/Croke, p.116; *The Morning Herald* newspaper, 15 May 1856, p.3
15. Goldie, p.253
16. Tastard, pp.101-2; Hinton (2019), p.117; *Medical & Surgical History*, v2, p.521
17. *Report of the Commissioners appointed to inquire into the regulations affecting the sanitary condition of the army*, v1, p.379, Question 10,020
18. Goldie, pp.244-5; Bolster, pp.264-5, *see* the letter in full pp.263-8
19. Bolster, pp.292, 296
20. Goldie, p.265
21. ODNB; Wyatt, pp.87,90; Wigglesworth, pp.4-5; Goldie, pp.265-71; Cook, v1 pp.299-301
22. Dossey, p.43; Bostridge, p.277; AB, II, pp.281-2
23. Dossey, p.43; Young, p.1698
24. Cook, v1, pp.296-7
25. Terrot, p.33
26. Goldie, p.218; Stanmore, v1, pp.418-19
27. Goldie, pp.244-5
28. Bostridge, pp.325-6
29. Dossey, p.40
30. Mackowiack (2007), pp.294-6
31. ODNB; Bostridge, pp.159, 281-2, 325-6; Cook, v1, pp.373; v2, pp.414-22

# BIBLIOGRAPHY

| | |
|---|---|
| AB | *Autobiography (Betsy Cadwaladyr)* |
| CClR | *Calendar of Close Rolls* |
| CPR | *Calendar of Patent Rolls* |
| CSP | *Dom Calendar of State Papers Domestic-Commonwealth 1652-1653, 1654, 1655* |
| DIB | *Dictionary of Irish Biography* |
| DWB | *Dictionary of Welsh Biography* |
| NLW | *National Library of Wales* |
| ODNB | *Oxford Dictionary of National Biography* |

## Online Sources

www.bl.ac.uk
www.britishnewspaperarchive.org.uk
www.clarelibrary.ie
https://daughtersofcharity.org/
https://discovery.nationalarchives.gov.uk
www.filles-de-la-charite.org
www.historic-shipping.co.uk
https://history.rcplondon.ac.uk (Dr Andrew Smith)
www.maritimearchives.co.uk (Lloyds List)
www.nam.ac.uk/explore/crimean-war
https://newspapers.library.wales/

*Bibliography*

https://nightingalesociety.com
www.papalencyclicals.net/councils (Church Councils)
www.rfsk.org.uk/history
https://sasra.org.uk (Scripture Readers)
https://search.lma.gov.uk/
www.sistersofmercy.ie
https://victorianweb.org/history/work/sullivan (Chapter 15)

## Articles & Unpublished Thesis Sources

'A Derbyshire Family' [article], Manuscripts and Special Collections, available at www.nottingham.ac.uk [accessed 2/8/22].

Barnard, L., (2017), *To what extent did the Royal Albert Asylum portray societal notions of 'idiots' and 'imbeciles' within the Victorin Era?* [thesis].

Bucknill, R.P., (2003), *Wherwell Abbey and its Cartulary,* London: King's College [thesis].

Clarke, A. (2016), 'The Execution of Sir Thomas More' [article], available at *Medieval Manuscripts Blog* www.blogs.bl.uk [accessed 23/9/22].

Cody, D. (2021), 'Social Class' [article], available at www.victorinaweb.org [accessed 5/5/23].

Collins, M. (2016), 'Remembering 20,000 Famine Refugees who died in 1847', *The Irish Times,* available at www.irishtimes.com [accessed 23/1/23].

Gregory, J., Dr (2020), 'Filthy Plymouth: An Environmental History of the Three Towns in the Nineteenth Century' [essay], University of Plymouth, available at filthy-plymouth.pdf (wordpress.com) [accessed 22/9/23].

'History of Lea Hurst - Nightingale's Derbyshire Home' [article], available at www.florencenightingale.org [accessed 2/8/22].

Hodkinson, R. (2022), 'Savoy Hospital' [article], available at www.lordgreys.weebly.com [accessed July 2022].

Huggon, M. (2018), *The Archaeology of the Medieval Hospital of England and Wales, 1066 – 1546,* University of Sheffield [thesis].

Jones, Gruffydd (2019), *The Incredible Adventures of Betsi Cadwaladr: 'Welsh Florence Nightingale' or 'Munchausen in Petticoats'? An evaluation of The Autobiography of Elizabeth Davis as a historical source,* The Open University: The making of Welsh history [dissertation].

Mackowiak, P. (2015), 'Florence Nightingale's syphilis that wasn't' [article], available from www.blog.oup.com [accessed 3/10/23].

Marrison, R. (2022), 'Class System in Victorian England' [article], available at www.HistoricalBritainBlog.com [accessed 5/5/23].

'Nightingale Family History' [article], available at www.lifeandtimesofflorencenightingale.wordpress.com [accessed 2/8/22].

Powell, E. (2018), *Spiritual Care Needs within an Assessment of Total Pain – the Challenges and Opportunities within a Community Setting,* [essay].

Redpath, A. (2018), 'Angélique Lucille Pringle: Florence Nightingale's favourite disciple' [article], available at www.thehistorygirlsscotland.com [accessed 12/8/23].

Riepel, L.M. (2017), *The Inherent Influence of Travel on an Emerging Feminist Icon: Florence Nightingale Abroad,* University of Central Oklahoma [thesis].

Ringlee, A.J. (2016), *THE ROMANOVS' MILITANT CHARITY: THE RED CROSS AND PUBLIC MOBILIZATION FOR WAR IN TSARIST RUSSIA, 1853-1914,* University of North Carolina [dissertation].

## Primary and Secondary Sources

AB – Williams, J. (1857) ed., *Betsy Cadwaladyr: a Balaclava Nurse: An Autobiography of Elizabeth Davis,* Honno: Welsh Women's Classics.

AMJ: Association Medical Journal (May 1855), *News and Topics of the Day* v3(125) pp.493-503, Published by: BMJ.

*Bibliography*

Abel-Smith, B. (1960), *A History of the Nursing Profession*, London: Heinmann, available at archive.org.

Army Medical Department (1858), *Medical and surgical history of the British Army: which served in Turkey and the Crimea during the war against Russia in the years 1854-55-56 Great Britain*, London: Harrison and Sons, available at http://resource.nlm.nih.gov/62510370R

Aloysius, M. Sister (1897), *Memories of the Crimea*, London: Burns & Oates Ltd.

Atkinson, J.C. (1879), *Cartularium abbathiae de Whiteby, Ordinis s. Benedicti, fundatae anno MLXXVIII*, Cartulary of Whitby Abbey, Volume 2, Durham: Andrews & Co., available at archive.org.

Bell, G. (1867), *Rough Notes by an Old Soldier, During fifty years' service, from Ensign G.B to Major-General, C.B.* Volumes I and II, London: Day, available at archive.org.

Bence-Jones, H. (1929), *An Autobiography* (with elucidations at later dates by his son, A. B. Bence-Jones), London: Crusha & Sons Ltd., available at archive.org [accessed 1/10/23].

Blomefield, F. (1860), *An Essay Towards a Topographical History of the County of Norfolk: Volume 4, the History of the City and County of Norwich, Part II*, available at British History Online.

Bloy, M. (2002), *The Light Cavalry Brigade in the Crimea: Extracts from the Letters and Journal of General Lord George Paget*, ed. John Murray (1881), available at https://victorianweb.org/history/crimea/paget/paget1.html

Bolster, E. (1964), *The Sisters of Mercy in the Crimean War*, Cork: The Mercier Press.

Bolton, J. L. (1980), *The Medieval English Economy 1150-1500*, London: Department of History Queen Mary College.

Bostock J.; Riley, H. (1857) eds., *The Natural History* by Pliny the Elder (77-79 CE), Volume 5, Book XXVIII, London: Bohn, available on archive.org.

Bostridge, M. (2009), *Florence Nightingale: the woman and her legend*, London: Viking.

Brayshay, M.; Pointon V.T. (1983), 'Local Politics and Public Health in mid-nineteenth century Plymouth', *Medical History* v27, pp.162-178.

Breay, M. (1897), 'Nursing in the Victorian Era', *The Nursing Record* v18(481), p.493. Royal College of Nursing Archives.

Briggs, A. (1984), *A Social History of England,* London: Book Club Associates.

Brown, A. (2018), 'The Forgotten Nurse of the Crimean War' [article], available at www.historyroom.org. [accessed 16/4/23].

Burfield, B. (2022), *Medieval Military Medicine: from the Vikings to the High Middle Ages*, Yorkshire: Pen & Sword.

Cantlie, N. (1974), *A History of the Army Medical Department, Volumes 1 and 2,* London: Churchill Livingstone.

Carlin, M. (1989), 'Medieval English Hospitals', in Granshaw, L.; Porter, R. (1989), *The Hospital in History,* London, New York: Routledge.

Carmoner, F.; Pereira, A.M.S. (2013), 'Herbal medicines: old and new concepts, truths and misunderstandings', *Brazilian Journal of Pharmacognosy* V23(2), pp.379-385.

Carpenter, D. (2015), *The cartulary of St Leonard's Hospital, York: Rawlinson volume I.* Publisher Woodbridge, Suffolk: Yorkshire Archaeological Society and the Borthwick Institute for Archives in association with the Boydell Press, available on archive.org.

Carroll, A. (1881), *Leaves from the Annals of the Sisters of Mercy in three volumes: I. Ireland. II. England, Scotland and the Colonies. III. America,* New York: The Catholic Publication Society Co.

Charaka-Samhita (2023), Chapter 9 and Chapter 15, available at www.carakasamhitaonline.com [accessed 2/10/22].

Clark, D. (2014), 'Total Pain: the work of Cicely Saunders and the maturing of a concept', *University of Glasgow: End of Life Studies* [Blog], available at http://endoflifestudies.academicblogs.co.uk [accessed 16/3/19].

Clarridge, A. (2018), 'Spirituality: A neglected aspect of care', in Chilton, S. and Bain, H. (2018), *A Textbook of Community Nursing*, Oxon: Routledge, pp.182 – 199.

*Bibliography*

Clay, R.M. (1909), *The Mediaeval Hospitals of England*, London: Methuen.

Colborne J.; Brine, F. (1857), *The Last of the Brave; or Resting Places of our Fallen heroes in the Crimea and at Scutari,* London: Ackermann and Co.

Connor, H. (1998), 'The use of chloroform by British Army Surgeons during the Crimean War', *Medical History,* v42(2), pp.161-193. See doi:10.1017/S0025727300063663

Conrad, L.I.; Neve, M.; Nutton, V.; Porter, R.; Wear, A. (1995), *The Western Medical Tradition 800 BC to AD 1800,* Cambridge University Press.

Cook, E. (1913), *The Life of Florence Nightingale. Volume 1 & II 1820 – 1910,* London: Macmillan & Co Ltd.

Cowen, R. (2006), *Relish: The Extraordinary Life of Alexis Soyer, Victorian Celebrity Chef.* London: Weidenfield & Nicolson.

Cullum, P. (1991), *Cremetts and Corrodies: care of the poor and sick at St Leonard's Hospital, York in the Middle Ages,* University of York.

Crumplin, M. (2018), 'Wellington's Combat Surgeon George James Guthrie' [article], available at www.waterlooassociation.org.uk [accessed 11/5/23].

Dickens, C. (2010), *Martin Chuzzlewit,* London: Vintage Classics.

Dock, L.; Stewart, I. (1920), *A Short History of Nursing: From the Earliest Times to the Present Day,* New York: Putnam & Sons.

Donohue, P. (1985), *Nursing: An Illustrated History,* Missouri: Mosby.

Doona, M.E. (1995), Sister Mary Joseph Croke: Another Voice from the Crimean War, 1854-1856, *Nursing History Review* v3 pp.3-41.

Dossey, B.M. (2010), 'Florence Nightingale: her Crimean Fever and Chronic Illness', *Journal of Holistic Nursing* V28(1), pp.38-53.

Doubleday, A.; Page, W. (1903), 'Houses of Benedictine nuns: Abbey of Wherwell', in *A History of the County of Hampshire* Volume 2, pp.132-137, available at British History Online [accessed 28/8/22].

Edwards, T.A. (2013), *The Art of Triage,* New York: Nova Sciences.

Ehrenreich, B.; English, D. (2010) 2nd ed., *Witches, Midwives & Nurses,* New York: Feminist Press.

Farmer, D.H. (2011), *The Oxford Dictionary of Saints,* New York: Oxford University Press.

Figes, O. (2011), *The Crimean War: A History,* London: Penguin.

First Commission (1855), *Report upon the state of the hospitals of the British army in the Crimea and Scutari, together with an appendix.* Contributors Great Britain. War Office. Royal College of Physicians of London, London: HMSO.

Fisher, G (2004), *The Crimean War 1854 – 1856,* Bristol Archives [pamphlet].

Fitzalan-Howard, H.G., Duke of Norfolk (1857), *The lives of Philip Howard, earl of Arundel, and of Anne Dacres, his wife,* London: Hurst & Blackett.

Frank, M. Sister (1953), *The Historical Development of Nursing,* London/Philadelphia: Saunders.

Gaweda, G. L. (2006), *The Transition from Monastic to Secular Medicine in Medieval England*, University of California [thesis].

Giles, J.A. (1847) ed., *William of Malmesbury's Chronicle of the Kings of England. From the earliest period to the reign of King Stephen*, London: Bohn.

Goldie, S. (1997), *Florence Nightingale: Letters from the Crimea,* Manchester: Mandolin.

Goytre Local History Group at http://www.goytrelocalhistory.org.uk/ [accessed 4/11/22].

Green, M. (2006), 'Getting to the Source: The Case of Jacoba Felicie and the Impact of the Portable Medieval Reader on the Canon of Medieval Women's History', *Medieval Feminist Forum* v42(1), pp.49-62.

Grignetti, F. (2022), *The Crimean War of the Daughters of Charity*, available at www.osservatoreromano.va [accessed 12/2/22].

Hagerty, J.M. (2004), 'A Catholic Chaplain in the Crimean War', *Journal of the Society for Army Historical Research* v82(329), pp.21-31, available at JSTOR [accessed 3/3/23].

Hamley, E.B. Sir (1891), *The War in the Crimea,* London: Seeley.

*Bibliography*

Hansard Archives, available at https://api.parliament.uk/historic-hansard/index.html

Haralambos, M.; Holborn, M. (2000), *Sociology: Themes and Perspectives,* LONDON: Collins Educational.

Helmstadter, C.; Godden, J. (2011), *Nursing Before Nightingale 1815 – 1899,* Surrey: Ashgate.

Helmstadter, C. (2020), *Beyond Nightingale: Nursing on the Crimean War battlefields,* Manchester University Press.

Hendriks, I.F.; Bovill, J.G.; Boer, F.; Houwaart E.S.; Hogendoorn, P.C.W. (2014), 'Nikolay Ivanovich Pirogov: a surgeon's contribution to military and civilian anaesthesia. *Anaesthesia* v70, pp.219–227, available at *doi:10.1111/anae.12916* [accessed 23/8/23].

Hendriks, I.F.; Zhuravlev, J.G.; Bovill, J.G.; Boer, F.; Hogendoorn, P.C.W. (2021), Women in healthcare in Imperial Russia: The contribution of the surgeon Nikolay I Pirogov', *Journal of Medical Biography* v19(1), pp.9-18. Chapter 6 at https://hdl.handle.net/1887/3491451

Hendriks, I.F. (2022), *Nikolay Ivanovich Pirogov and his contribution to medicine in 19th Century Imperial Russia,* retrieved from https://hdl.handle.net/1887/3491451

Hilton, L. (2008), *Queens Consort: England's Medieval Queens,* London: Weidenfeld & Nicolson.

Hinton, M. (2015), 'Reporting the Crimean War: Misinformation and Misinterpretation', *Interdisciplinary Studies in the Long Nineteenth Century* v20, pp.1-19.

Hinton, M. (2019), *Victory over Disease: Resolving the medical crisis in the Crimean War, 1854-1856,* Warwick: Helion & Co.

Historic England *Disability in Medieval Hospitals and Almshouses,* available at https://historicengland.org.uk/ [accessed 23/1/23].

Howard, J.; Bailey, J.B. (1884), *The condition of gaols, hospitals, and other institutions,* Royal College of Surgeons of England, London: H.K. Lewis.

Huntsman, R.G.; Bruin, M.; Holttum, D. (2002), 'Twixt Candle and Lamp: The Contribution of Elizabeth Fry and the Institution of

Nursing Sisters to Nursing Reform', *Medical History*, v46, pp.351-380. Cambridge University Press.

Hunter, Rev (1834), *An Introduction to the Valor Ecclesiasticus of King Henry VIII,*

Hurd-Mead, K. (1938), *A history of women in medicine, from the earliest times to the beginning of the nineteenth century,* The Haddam Press.

Institution for Nursing Sisters (1848), *Report of the Institution for Nursing Sisters, No. 16, Broad Street Buildings, Bishopsgate: Established 1840,* London: Teape.

Jameson, A. (1857), *Sisters of Charity, Catholic and Protestant. And the communion of labor,* Boston: Ticknor and Fields.

Jameson, A. (1890), *Legends of the Monastic Orders as represented in the Fine Arts,* London: Longman Green.

Jessopp, A.; James, M.R (1896) ed., *The life and miracles of St. William of Norwich by Thomas of Monmouth,* Cambridge University Press.

Jonsen, A.R. (2000), *A Short History of Medical Ethics,* New York: Oxford University Press.

Jones, W.H.S. (1909), *Malaria and Greek History,* Manchester: University Press.

Jones, M. (1960), *Elizabeth Davies, 1789-1860,* Cardiff: University of Wales Press.

Kinglake, A.W. (1902), *Invasion of the Crimea: Its origin, and account of its progress down to the death of Lord Raglan,* Volume 7.

Kleisiaris C.F.; Sfakianakis C.; Papathanasiou I.V. (2014), 'Healthcare Practices in Ancient Greece: The Hippocratic Ideal', *Journal of Medical Ethics and History of Medicine* v7(6), available at https://pubmed.ncbi.nlm.nih.gov/25512827/

Knowles, D. (1963), *The Monastic Order in England; A history of its development from the times of St. Dunstan to the Fourth Lateran Council, 940-1216,* Cambridge University Press.

Kyle, R.A. (2001), 'Historical Review – Henry Bence Jones – Physician, Chemist, Scientist and Biographer: A Man for All Season.', *British Journal of Haematology* v115, pp.13-18.

*Bibliography*

Lane-Poole, S. (1888), *The Life of the Right Honourable Stratford Canning, Viscount Stratford de Redcliffe* in two volumes, London New York: Longmans, Green & Co.

Lawson, G. (1858), *On gunshot wounds of the thorax and the treatment pursued for them in the Crimea, contrasted with that which was followed in former campaigns*, London: Born.

Leduc, G. (2005), 'Women in the Army in Eighteenth Century Britain', in Baudino, I.; Carré, J.; Révauger, eds. (2005), *Invisible Women*, Oxon: Routledge. See Chapter 6.

Lindgrén, S.; Neumann, J. (1980), 'Great Historical Events that were Significantly Affected by the Weather: 5, Some Meteorological Events of the Crimean War and Their consequences', *American Meteorological Society* v61(12) pp.1570-1583.

*Lloyd's List* (1813-1814), available at Hathi Trust [accessed 15/2/23].

Lost Hospitals of London, available at https://ezitis.myzen.co.uk/florencenightingale.html [accessed 22/5/19].

Luddy, M. (2004), *The Crimean Journals of the Sisters of Mercy 1854-56,* Dublin: Four Courts Press.

Lysons, D. (1795), 'Marylebone', in *The Environs of London: Volume 3, County of Middlesex*, pp.242-279, available at http://www.british-history.ac.uk/london-environs/vol3/pp242-279 [accessed 8/10/23].

MacDonald, I. (1935), 'Elizabeth Alkin: A Florence Nightingale of the Commonwealth', *British Journal of Nursing* v83, p.119.

Mackowiak, P. (2007), *Post mortem: solving history's great medical mysteries,* Philadelphia, Penn: American College of Physicians.

Manwaring, G.E. (1936), *The Flower of England's Garden,* London: Philip Alan.

Marrison, R. (2022), *Class System in Victorian England,* available at https://historicalbritainblog.com/ [accessed 23/1/23].

Maslow, A. H. (1943), 'A theory of human motivation', *Psychological Review*, v50(4), pp.370–396. See https://doi.org/10.1037/h0054346 [accessed 23/10/22].

Maxwell, P.B. (1855), *Whom shall we hang? The Sebastopol inquiry*, London: James Ridgway.

McDonald, L. (2014), 'Florence Nightingale and Irish nursing', *Journal of Clinical Nursing* v23, pp.2424-2433.

Meehan, T. (2003), 'Careful nursing: a model for contemporary nursing practice', *Journal of Advanced Nursing* v44(1), pp.99-107.

Meehan, T. (2012), 'The Careful Nursing philosophy and professional practice model', *Journal of Clinical Nursing* v21, pp.2905-2916.

Millengen, J. (1819), *The army medical officer's manual upon active service, or, Precepts for his guidance in the various situations in which he may be placed: with observations on the preservation of the health of armies upon foreign service,* London: Burgess and Hill.

Minkowski, W.L. (1992), 'Women Healers of the Middle Ages: Selected Aspects of Their History', *American Journal of Public Health* v82(2) pp.288-295.

Mitra, S.M. (1911), *The life and letters of Sir John Hall*, London, New York: Longmans, Green and Co.

More, T. (1516), *UTOPIA & Selected Epigrams.* Editors Wegemer, G.B; Smith, S.W; Translated by Malsbary, G; Ritter, B; Young, C, Ellis, E (2020), University of Dallas: CTMS.

Mount, T. (2016), *Medieval Medicine: Its Mysteries and Science,* Stroud: Amberley.

Murphy-Hiscock, A. (2017), T*he Green Witch: Your Complete Guide to the Natural Magic of Herbs, Flowers, Essential Oils and more,* New York: Simon & Schuster.

National Archives Ireland (2015), *Survey of Hospital Archives in Ireland,* v7 at https://www.nationalarchives.ie [accessed 3/11/22].

Nightingale, F. (1851), *The Institution of Kaiserswerth on the Rhine, for the Practical Training of Deaconesses, under the direction of the Rev. Pastor Fliedner, embracing the Support and Care of a Hospital, Infant and Industrial schools, and a Female Penitentiary,* London Ragged Colonial Training School.

Nightingale, F. (1858), *Notes on matters affecting the health, efficiency, and hospital administration of the British Army: founded chiefly on the experience of the late war,* London: Harrison.

*Bibliography*

Nightingale, F. (1859), *Notes on Nursing,* New York: Dover (1969 reprint).

Nightingale, F. (1863), *Notes on Hospitals,* London: Longman, Roberts and Green.

Nolan, W. (1786), *An essay on humanity: or a View of Abuses in Hospitals with a plan for correcting them,* London: Murray, Fleet Street.

'Nurses and Doctors: Systems of Nursing, By A Nurse' (1880), *Edinburgh Medical Journal* v25(11) pp.1048-1052.

Nutting, A.; Dock, L. (1907), *A History of Nursing Volume 1 - 4.* New York: Putnam & Sons.

O'Malley, I.B. (1931), *Florence Nightingale 1820- 1856: A study of her life down to the end of the Crimean War,* London: Thornton & Butterworth Ltd.

Page, W. (1906) ed., 'Hospitals: Holy Innocents without Lincoln', in *A History of the County of Lincoln:* v2, pp.230-232, available at British History Online [accessed 26/2/23].

Page, W. (1909), 'Hospitals: Hospital of the Savoy', in *A History of the County of London: Volume 1, London Within the Bars, Westminster and Southwark.* v1, pp.546-549. British History Online [accessed 26/2/23].

Page, W. (1974) ed., 'Hospitals: York', in *A History of the County of York.* v3, pp.336-352, available at British History Online. [accessed 13/1/23].

Penney, M.E. (1954), 'Letters from Therapia, 1855', *Blackwood's Magazine* v275(1663), pp.413-421.

Peterkin, A.; Johnston, W.; Drew, R. (1907), *Commissioned officers in the medical services of the British Army, 1660-1960,* London: Wellcome Historical Medical Library.

Power, E. (1926), 'The Position of Women', in *The Legacy of the Middle Ages,* ed. Crump, C.; Jacob, E., Oxford Uni Press.

Power, E. (1975) ed., Postan (1997), *Medieval Women,* Cambridge University Press.

Ralls, W. (1974), 'The Papal Aggression of 1850: A Study in Victorian Anti-Catholicism', *Church History* v43(2), pp.242-256.

Rappaport, H. (2007), *No Place for Ladies: the untold story of women in the Crimea,* London: Aurum.

Rawcliffe, C. (1995), *The hospitals of medieval Norwich,* Centre of East Anglian Studies, University of East Anglia.

Rawcliffe, C. (1996), *Sources for the History of Medicine in late Medieval England,* Michigan: Teams.

Rawcliffe, C. (1997), *Medicine and Society in Later Medieval England,* Stroud: Sutton.

Rawcliffe, C. (2002), "'Written in the Book of Life': The libraries of medieval English hospitals and almshouses', *The Library* v3(2) pp.127-162.

Reid, D.A., Dr (1911), *Memories of the Crimean War, January 1855 to June 1856,* London: St Catherine Press.

Reports of the Commissioners of Inquiry into the State of Education in Wales (1848), *In Three Parts: Part I Carmarthen, Glamorgan and Pembroke, Part II Brecknock, Cardigan, Radnor and Monmouth, Part III North Wales,* London: HMSO.

Report of the Commissioners (1858), appointed to inquire into the regulations affecting the sanitary condition of the army, the organization of military hospitals, and the treatment of the sick and wounded: *with evidence and appendix [Vol. 1].* Contributors: Great Britain – Royal Commission Appointed to Inquire Into the Sanitary Condition of the Army. Nightingale, Florence, 1820-1910. Herbert, Sidney, Sir, 1810-1861; St. Thomas's Hospital Medical School Library; King's College London, London: Eyre & Spottiswoode for H.M.S.O.

Report of the Commissioners (1858), appointed to inquire into the regulations affecting the sanitary condition of the army, the organization of military hospitals, and the treatment of the sick and wounded: *Appendix LXXIX [Vol. 2].* Contributors: Great Britain - Royal Commission Appointed to Inquire Into the Sanitary Condition of the Army; Herbert of Lea, Sidney Herbert, Baron, 1810-1861. Royal College of Physicians of London, London: Eyre & Spottiswoode for H.M.S.O.

## Bibliography

'Register of Nurses Sent to the Military Hospitals in the East', available at Florence Nightingale Museum here: Register-of-Nurses.pdf (florence-nightingale.co.uk) [accessed 10/10/22].

Roberts, G.T. (2019), Davis, Elizabeth (Betsi Cadwaladr) (1789-1860), nurse and traveller. *DWB*.

Rogers, J. (1889), *Reminiscence of a Workhouse Medical Officer*, London: Unwin.

Rosedahl, C.; Kowalski, M. (2007) 9th ed., *Textbook of Basic Nursing*, Lippincott, Williams & Wilkins.

Roxburgh, R. (1969), 'Miss Nightingale and Miss Clough; Letters from the Crimea', *Victorian Studies* v13(1) pp.71-89, available at www.jstor.org [accessed March 2023].

Rubin, M. (1989), 'Development and change in English hospitals', in Granshaw, L.; Porter, R. (1989), *The Hospital in History*, London, New York: Routledge.

Russell, W.H. (1858), *The British Expedition to the Crimea*, London: Routledge.

Sabatini, S. (1994), 'Women, Medicine and Life in the Middle Ages (500 – 1500 AD)', *American Journal of Nephrology* v14 pp.391-8.

Sams, S. (2015), 'Dominique Jean Larrey – Surgeon in Chief of Napoleon's Armies', *Royal College of Surgeons of England*, available at www.rcseng.ac.uk [accessed 24/8/23].

Saunderson, R. (1836), *Ychydig gofnodau am fywyd a marwolaeth Dafydd Cadwaladr.*

Shepherd, J. (1991), *The Crimean Doctors: A History of the British Medical Services in the Crimean War. Volume I & II,* Liverpool University Press.

Skandalakis, P.N.; Lainas, P.; Zoras, O.; Skandalakis, J.E.; Mirilas, P. (2006), 'To Afford the Wounded Speedy Assistance: Dominique Jean Larrey and Napoleon', *World Journal of Surgery.* v30 pp.1392–1399.

Smith, W. (1870) ed., *Dictionary of Greek and Roman Biography and Mythology.*

Sorokina, T. S. (1995), 'Russian nursing in the Crimean war', *Journal of the Royal College of Physicians of London* v29(1) pp.57-63

Soyer, A. (1857), *Soyer's Culinary Campaign: Being Historical Reminiscences of the Late War. With the Plain Art of Cookery for Military and Civil Institutions, the Army, Navy, Public etc, etc*, London: G. Routledge & Co.

Stanmore, A.H-G. (1906), *Sidney Herbert, Lord Herbert of Lea: A Memoir*, London: Murray.

Stell, P. (1996), *Medieval Practice in Medieval York*, University of York, Borthwick Paper No.90.

Sullivan, M.C. (1995), *Catherine McAuley and the tradition of mercy*, University of Notre Dame Press.

Summers, A. (1989), 'The Mysterious Demise of Sarah Gamp: The Domiciliary Nurse and Her Detractors, c. 1830-1860', *Victorian Studies* v32(3) pp.365-386. Indiana University Press.

Swift, R. (1987), 'The Outcast Irish in the British Victorian City: Problems and Perspectives', *Irish Historical Studies* v24(99), pp.264-276.

Tastard, T. (2023), *Nightingale's Nuns and the Crimean War*, London: Bloomsbury Academic

Taylor, F. (1857) 3rd ed., *Eastern Hospitals and English Nurses: The narrative of twelve months' experience in the hospitals of Koulali and Scutari*, London: Hurst & Blackett.

Terrot, S.A. (1898), *Reminiscences of Scutari Hospitals in winter 1854-55*, Edinburgh: Stevenson.

The British Medical Journal (1897), *The Nursing of the Sick under Queen Victoria.* v1, pp.1644-1648.

*The Churchman's Companion* (August 1849), Part 32, v6, pp.108-110.

*The Churchman's Companion* (April 1849), Part 28, v5, pp.243-8.

*The Home-life of English Ladies in the XVII Century* (1860), Anon, London: Bell & Daldy.

The Irish Monthly Journal (1892) *Joanna Reddan* v20(227), pp.225-236, available at https://www.jstor.org/stable/20498358 [accessed 3/3/23].

*The Manuscripts of His Grace the Duke of Portland, preserved at Welbeck Abbey* (1891), London: HMSO.

## Bibliography

*The Medical and Surgical History of the British Army which Served in Turkey and the Crimea During the War Against Russia in the Years 1854-55-56:* Volume 1 & II. 1858, London: HMSO, available at https://collections.nlm.nih.gov/catalog/nlm:nlmuid-62510370R-mvset

Thorp, D.J. (2015), *Betsi Cadwaladr: A Welsh Nurse in the Crimea*, Kindle.

Twining, L. (1866), *A Letter to the President of the Poor Law Board on Workhouse Infirmaries.*

Twining, L. (1898), *Workhouses and pauperism and women's work in the administration of the Poor law.*

Tyler, A. (2001), 'Lord Palmerston and the Irish Famine Emigration', *The Historical Journal, 44, 2 (2001)*, pp.441-469. Open Access at Centre for Economic Research Working Paper Series, No. WP01/19, University College Dublin, Department of Economics, Dublin, https://hdl.handle.net/10197/1318

Usherwood, C. (1852 – 1856), Service Journal available at https://victorianweb.org/history/crimea/usher/usherov.html [accessed 11/12/22].

Verney, H. (1970), *Florence Nightingale at Harley Street: her reports to the governors of her nursing home 1853-4,* London: Dent & Sons.

Wakely, E.; Carson, J. (2011), 'Historical recovery heroes – Florence Nightingale', *Mental Health and Social Inclusion*, v15(1), pp.24-28.

Walcott, M. (1868), 'Inventories of (I) St Mary's Hospital of Maison Dieu Dover (II.) The Benedictine Priory of St Martin New-Work Dover for Monks (III) The Benedictine Priory of St Mary and St Sexburge in the Island of Sheppey for Nuns', *Archaeologia Cantiana.* Volume 7: pp.272-306, available at www.kentarchaeology.org.uk.

Walsh, J. (1911), *Old-Time Makers of Medicine,* New York: University Press.

Waters, C. (1999), *A Dictionary of Old Trades, Titles and Occupations,* Newbury: Countryside Books.

White, R. (1978), *Social change and the development of the nursing profession: a study of the Poor law nursing service 1848-1948,* London: Kimpton.

White, E. (2014), 'Improving conditions for the wounded: Dominique Jean Larrey', *Wounds UK.* v10(4), p114.

White, M. (2009), *The Industrial Revolution: Georgian Britain* [article], available at www.bl.uk [accessed 17/2/23]

W.H.O - World Health Organisation (2019), Traditional, Complementary and Integrative Medicine, available at www.who.int

Wigglesworth, G. (2010), *Florence Nightingale's Journey Home from the Crimea,* available at www.wigglesworth.me.uk/local_history [accessed 3/10/23].

Wilkinson, L.J. (2020), *The Household Roll of Eleanor de Montfort, Countess of Leicester and Pembroke, 1265,* Suffolk: The Pipe Roll Society, Boydell Press.

Williams, T.J. (1947), 'The Beginnings of Anglican Sisterhoods', *Historical Magazine of the Protestant Episcopal Church, English Church History Number II* v16(4) pp.350-372.

Williams, K. (2008), 'Reappraising Florence Nightingale', *British Medical Journal* Volume 337(2889), pp.1461-1463

Windham, C (1897), *The Crimean diary and letters of Lieut.-General Sir Charles Ash Windham, K.C.B: with observations upon his services during the Indian mutiny, and an introduction by Sir William Howard Russell*, ed. Hugh Pease. London: Kegan Paul, Trench, Trübner & Co Ltd.

Woodham-Smith, C. (1951), *Florence Nightingale: 1820-1910*, New York: McGraw-Hill

Wrottesley, G (1898) *Crecy and Calais.* London: HMO.

Wyatt L. (2019), *A History of Nursing*, Stroud: Amberley Publishing.

Young, D.A.B. (1995), Florence Nightingale's Fever, *British Medical Journal* Volume 311, pp.1697-1700.

*Yr Haul* (May 1878), No.257, NLW, available in the Welsh language at https://journals.library.wales/view/2785689.

# Index

Alkin, Elizabeth, 27-9
Almshouse, 7, 11, 13, 23, 69
Anglican Sisterhood, 45-6
   Sellon, Lydia, 46
   Terrot, Anne, 51, 109, 120, 138
Ambulance Corps, 35, 89, 90-2
Army Chaplains, 81, 84
Army Medical Service, 32, 34, 86-7, 91, 123
   *also* Commissariat Dept, 52, 79, 85-6, 125
Asylums, 23, 54-5, 69, 74

Baggott Street Convent, Dublin, 44-5, 99
Balaklava, 33, 48, 52, 119, 129, 134
   Hospital – Castle, 123, 128, 138
   Hospital – General, 110, 113, 115-6, 118, 121-3, 126, 128, 131-2, 135-7, 139
Battle of Alma, 34-5, 62, 122

Battle of Waterloo, 39, 82, 90-1
Bence Jones, Dr Henry, 72-3
Bracebridge, Charles, viii, 68, 70, 96-8, 105, 113
   *Also* Selina, 68-9, 95-7, 115-6
Bridgeman, Mary Francis, vii-xv, 38, 42, 45, 51
   Pre-Crimea, 53-7
   Nursing in the Crimea, 79, 82, 92, 96-8, 100, 102-05, 109, 114, 117-19, 122-3, 126-7, 139
   Post-Crimea, 130-36
   *See also* Reddan, Joanna, xiv, 54-5, 57

Cadwaladyr, Betsy, vii-xv, 41, 51
   Pre-Crimea, 58-63
   Nursing in the Crimea, 79, 85, 92, 96-8, 101-02, 104-05, 107, 109-10, 113, 115-17, 121-3, 125, 127

Post-Crimea, 128-9, 130
*Also* Bridget (sister), xiv, 61-3, 101, 130
Campbell, Sir John (Brigadier General of the Highland Brigade), 42
Careful Nursing Philosophy, ix-xii, 44, 55-6
Catholic/Catholicism, x, 8, 17-19, 25, 45-6, 68, 80-4, 87, 95-6, 99, 100, 105, 117, 132, 134
Cholera, ix, 26, 31-2, 34-5, 42, 47, 50, 50-1, 54-7, 76, 90, 92-3, 99, 114, 121, 124, 132
Clough, Martha, 41-2, 89, 116
Codrington, Sir William, General, 133
Colic, 120
Constantinople, viii, 31, 42, 45, 77-8, 90, 93, 96, 98, 100, 102, 104-05, 117, 136
Crimean Fever, 138

**Crimean War Doctors**
Anderson, Dr Arthur, 121
Beatson, Dr George, 131
Brett, Dr Frederick, 90
Dumbreck, Dr David, 88, 93, 124
Lawson, Dr George, 34, 50
Menzies, Dr Duncan, 76, 125

O'Connor, Dr Nicholas, 118-9
Spence, Dr Thomas, 52, 121

**Crimean War and Passenger Ships**
*The Calcutta* (took Betsy home from Crimea), 129
*The Cleopatra* (took Sisters of Mercy home from Crimea), 133-4
*The Danube* (took Nightingale home), 136
*The Egypt* (took Betsy and Bridgeman to Crimea), 102
*The Melbourne* (took Betsy from Scutari Hospital to Balaklava), 116
*The Prince* (supply ship lost in the Great Storm), 51-2, 121
*The Resolute* (supply ship lost in the Great Storm), 52

Daughters of Charity, 27, 31, 36-7, 96
Deaconesses, 69, 70
Depression, 67, 97, 139, 140
Diarrhoea, 51, 118, 120-1, 127, Appendix 2
Dickens, Charles, xii, 21-3, 25 *See* Gamp, Sarah, 102

*Index*

Dublin, xi, xiii, 43-5, 82, 99
Dunne, Colonel, 31, 85
Dysentery, 31, 51, 93, 113-4, 120, 128

Establishment for Gentlewomen during Temporary Illness, 41, 71-3
Extra-diet kitchens, 63, 109-10, 113-14, 117, 126

Fever, 15, 32, 57, 93, 113, 118, 120-21, 137-39
Flying Ambulance, 38-9
Frostbite, 26, 49, 118, 121, 135
Fry, Elizabeth, 71

Gamp, Sarah (fictional), *see* Dickens, Charles
Great Irish Famine, ix, 56-7, 80, 86, 111
Great Storm, 48, 51, 121
    *Also* Hurricane, xiv, 48-9

Hall, Dr John, xv, 38, 50, 87, 123, 129, 135
Harley Street, 41, 73-7, 96-7
Helena, Empress (Ancient Rome), 3
Helena, Grand Duchess (Russia), 39
Herbert, Sidney, viii, 41, 44, 64, 68, 72, 76-7, 81-2, 86, 88, 92-3, 95, 97, 99-100, 104, 109, 116-18, 126, 139
Hildegard of Bingen, 14
Hippocrates, x, 2
Hospital Marquees, 50, 93, 121
Hurricane *see* Great Storm

Kaiserswerth, 69-70, 73
    *Also* Fliedner, Pastor Theodore, 69, 70
Kinsale Convent, 44-5, 56-7, 134, 136
Koulali, 83, 113, 117, 122-3, 128, 138, Appendix 2
    Hospital – Barrack, 118-9
    Hospital – General, 118-9

Lady Llanover, Augusta Hall, 62, 101-02
Lady Maria Forester, 76-7
Lady Nurse ix, xii, 41, 43, 97
Lady Superintendents of Nursing, 41, 46, 71, 73, 123
Larrey, Dominique Jean (Napoleon's Military Field Surgeon), 38-9
    *See also* Triage
**London Hospitals**
    Guys, 63, 72, 123
    Middlesex, 76, 107
    St Bart's, 20, 85
    St George's, 72, 100
    St Thomas', 72, 123

Lord Palmerston (Prime Minister from 1855), 66, 76-7, 85
Lord Raglan (Field Marshal), 31, 35, 42, 63, 89, 112-13, 116, 123, 125-26

Malnutrition, 110
McAuley, Catherine, ix – xi, 43-4, 55
McKenzie, Eliza (Naval Nurse), xv, 106-07
Medical Dressers, 119, 135
Medical Staff Corps, 92
Monasteries, xi, 3, 5-6, 8, 16-17
Moore, Mother Superior M. Clare, 44-5, 56, 114, 117, 132

Nightingale, Florence, vii – xv, 13, 23, 25, 29-30, 34, 37-8, 41-8, 51, 57
   Childhood and Pre-Crimea, 64-78
   Nursing in Crimea, 79-80, 82-8, 90, 92, 94-101, 104-06, 109-14, 119, 125
   *With Betsy*, 58-9, 62, 105, 115-17, 128-29
   *With Bridgeman*, 57, 59, 62, 105, 117-18, 130-35
   Post-Crimea and Illness, 136-141
   Parthenope, 66, 98, 137
   William, 66

*Noblesse Oblige,* 41, 76
Nunneries, 6, 16
Nurse Register (details of nurses sent to Crimea), 101-02, 117
Nurse Selection for Crimea, 98-9

Orderlies, viii, 26, 34, 77, 84, 87, 90, 92-4, 109, 118-19, 122, 135
Orphanages, 18, 55, 69
Ottoman Empire, 29

Paris, 16, 36, 44-45, 61, 70, 73, 81, 95-6, 102, 130, 137
Parliament Joan *see* Alkin, Joan
Pauper Nurse, 24-5
Pelham-Clinton, Sir Henry (5th Duke of Newcastle), 40, 86, 88-9, 91
Pirogov, Nikolay, 37-40
Plymouth, 46-7
Portsmouth, 28, 47, 129, 134
Poultices, ix, 3, 10, 55, 122, 124
Poverty, xiv, 1, 6, 13, 20, 54, 56, 62, 85, 129-130, 136, 141
Proselytism, 82-3
Protestant, 19, 68-9, 72, 81-4, 95, 117

Reformation, x, 17, 19-20, 46, 80

## Index

Renaissance, 17, 19-20
Roberts, Eliza, xiv, 113
Ronan, Father William (Catholic priest of the Sisters of Mercy), 83-4, 100, 117, 123
Russell, William Howard, 33, 35, 62
Russia, vii, 29-31, 35, 37, 39-40, 49, 118

Salerno Medical School, 15
Sanitation, 73, 121, 124, 141
Saunders, Dame Cicely, x
Savoy Palace, 27
Sebastopol, 31, 38, 112
Scurvy, 32, 49
Scutari, xiv, 26, 34, 37, 63, 76-8, 88, 92, 94, 100, 104-05, 108, 111, 113, 118-9, 123-25, 128, 131, 135, 138, Appendix 2
   *See* Hospital – Barrack, 114-15, 117-9, 120, 124
   *See* Hospital – General, 109, 114, 117-8
Sisters of Mercy – Irish, vii, ix, x, xi, xii, xiii, xiv, 30, 42, 48, 138-9
   Pre-Crimea, 43-5, 54-7
   Nursing in Crimea, 80, 82-4, 92, 95-6, 98-100, 102-03, 105, 114, 117-8, 122, 127
   Post-Crimea, 130-32, 134-36
   *See also* Doyle, Aloysius, xii, xiii, 43, 83, 99, 103, 105, 109, 114, 118, 131-2
   *See also* Croke, Mary Joseph, xii, 131-2, 134
Sisters of Mercy – Russia, 37, 39
Smith, Andrew Dr, viii, xv, 30, 32, 52, 76, 87-93, 113, 121, 124-5
Stanley, Mary, 41-3, 58, 68, 83, 95-6, 101-03, 105, 107-08, 118
Soyer, Alexis, 110-113, 137
St Fabiola, 3
St Hilde of Whitby, 6
St John's House (lay Sisterhood and nurse training school), 23, 46-7, 96, 104
St Leonard's Medieval Hospital, York, 9-10
St Marcella, 3-4
St Paula, 3

Taylor, Fanny (Frances), xii, ixv, 97, 102-03, 105-06, 108, 111, 120
Therapia, 104-08, 114, 116, 118, 138
Triage, 37-9
Twining, Louisa, 23, 41

Varna, 31-5, 124-5

War Office, viii, 72, 82-4, 90, 94, 98-101, 104, 110, 117, 124, 132
Wherwell Abbey, 10-11
Whitby Abbey, 6
Workhouse, 23-5, 57, 85, 97

Wound/Wounded/Wounds, vii, xiv, 10, 12, 15-16, 26, 28, 30-32, 34-5, 37-41, 49-50, 63, 86, 114, 119-20, 122-3, 133, 135